HERBS
AND
HERB LORE
OF
COLONIAL AMERICA

Colonial Dames of America

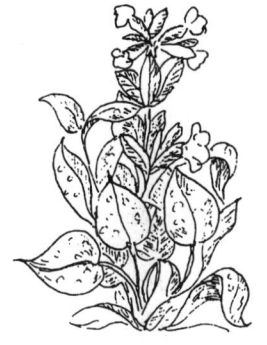

DOVER PUBLICATIONS, INC.
New York

Published in Canada by General Publishing Company, Ltd., 30 Lesmill Road, Don Mills, Toronto, Ontario.

Bibliographical Note

This Dover edition, first published in 1995, is an unabridged republication of the work originally published in 1970 under the title *Simples, Superstitions & Solace: Plant Material Used in Colonial Living*, with the title-page credit "Compiled by the Grounds Committee of the National Society of the Colonial Dames of America in the State of Connecticut." In the main part of the book, the illustrations were originally on separate pages; in the Dover edition they have been combined with the corresponding text.

Library of Congress Cataloging-in-Publication Data

Simples, superstitions & solace

    Herbs and herb lore of colonial America / Colonial Dames of America.

       p.   cm.

    Originally published: Simples, superstitions & solace. Wethersfield, Conn. : Grounds Committee of the National Society of the Colonial Dames of America in the State of Connecticut. 1970.

    Includes bibliographical references (p.   ) and index.

    ISBN 0-486-28529-4 (pbk.)

    1. Herbs—New England—History. 2. Plants, Useful—New England—History. 3. Herbs—Therapeutic use—New England—History. 4. Plants—Folklore—History. 5. Folklore—New England—History. 6. New England—History—To 1775. I. Colonial Dames of America. II. Title.

SB351.H5S576   1995

581.6'3'0974—dc20   94-48527

                                                          CIP

Manufactured in the United States of America
Dover Publications, Inc., 31 East 2nd Street, Mineola, N.Y. 11501

. . . a certain shepherd lad
Of small regard to see, yet well skill'd
In every virtuous plant, and healing herb

                    . . .

. . . would beg me sing:
Which, when I did, he on the tender grass
Would sit, and hearken even to ecstasy,
And in requital ope his leathern scrip,
And show me Simples, of a thousand names,
Telling their strange and vigorous faculties.

JOHN MILTON, *Comus*

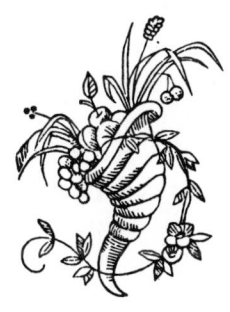

Introduction

Plant material used in Colonial gardens reveals unexpected insights into the life of the times. The restorations of houses recreate early kitchens, charming parlors, bedrooms, and other rooms where we can picture the activities of the housewife and her family. The garden, however, tells us what was needed to sustain pioneer life when land was the source of supply with each square foot carefully put to various useful purposes. This little volume is an attempt to share with the reader the enchantment which abounds in the study of early horticulture.

Without long days of arduous labor and the careful utilization of the bounty which nature provided, survival would have been impossible. Without faith in their own simple knowledge of life, courage might have failed and spirits broken. In working with the Colonial Dames' land in Wethersfield, Connecticut, great care is being exercised in surrounding the three adjacent eighteenth-century houses with the plant material and general land usage which made life possible for the colonists of the period. Dwarf fruit trees are planted among utilitarian plants and a scattering of flowers. Large sections are generally broken into small beds, or planting areas, while clipped and spacious lawns should be nonexistent. All plant material is being carefully researched and documented as being available in New England prior to the nineteenth century.

Early herbals facilitate the identification of plants for medicinal purposes. They were the precursors of the science of medicine; and the knowledge which these books dispensed was of utmost importance. Although the earliest book originated around the Mediterranean and was attributed to Hippocrates, the first written in English, Bankes' *Herball,* was published in London in 1525. There followed immediately several herbals of major importance. The first to be illustrated was the *Greate Herball* published in 1526. An important book by John Gerard was introduced in 1597. This volume was laced with anecdotes, legends, and fables, which were usually presented as facts. John Gerard was a physician and gardener as well as the superintendent of Lord Burleigh's two gardens and his opinions and instructions received serious attention. Thus many fantastic superstitions were given strict credence by the populace of the day and were handed down from generation to generation. When the science of medicine developed, herbals were no longer considered vital to survival.

American colonists, however, journeying into remote areas, brought with them from their homelands much of this lore. This they augmented with information gleaned from the Indians on the use of native plants which proved invaluable to them.

The use of herbs and other available plants fell into many categories. Often each one was credited with a myriad of interchangeable properties. These were of great importance in the kitchen. As medicines they were often all that was available to the early settlers, therefore irreplaceable. As natural dyes, they added color to lives of primitive deprivation, and in many cases helped to make life bearable under difficult conditions of living. Sanitation and refrigeration were relatively unknown. Thus the strewing of herbs for fragrance and disinfection was a common practice. Meat seasoned with herbs became more palatable. All of these uses required infinite patience. Plants were grown, harvested, preserved, and stored, and then the concoctions were carefully prepared.

Webster's *Dictionary* defines a "simple" as "a medicinal plant, each vegetable being supposed to possess a virtue and to constitute a simple remedy." Strokes, heart disease, fevers, colic, and gout were only a few of the miseries susceptible to almost magical cures by "simples."

We are familiar with the word "superstition," and all that it implies of fearful imagination and prayerful hope. After tumultuous and dangerous Atlantic crossings into a wilderness of Indians and beasts of the forest, superstitions, as defined in the ancient herbals, must have given many a delicate lady the courage to face her new life.

How great the need of solace in a strange and alien world, fraught with danger and hardships! Every precious bit of home was cherished and nurtured by the gallant women. Not the least of their memories of home was often recreated by slips and seeds of plants tucked into their meager luggage. Their very lives depended on medicinal herbs, while an occasional rose for beauty brought joy and solace to their hearts.

Fruit Trees

Apple, Pear, Peach, and Cherry

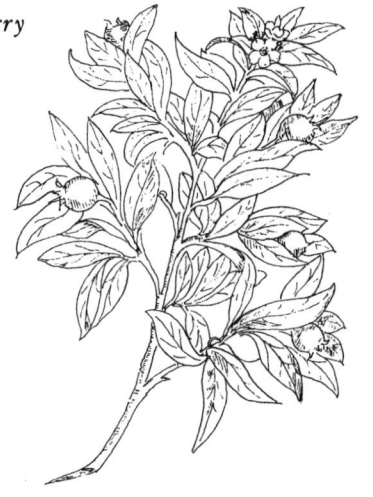

Medlar

The medlar apple chosen for this illustration dates from 1565. According to Blackwell's *A Curious Herbal*, written in 1739, medlars were "esteemed cooling and drying and binding especially before they are quite ripe and are useful in all kinds of fluxes. Some commend the hard seed as good for ye gravel and stone." This tree is still obtainable and was planted recently in Wethersfield with Belle et Bonne, an old Connecticut apple. Also planted were Black Gilliflower, another eighteenth-century apple, McClellan, which originated in Woodstock in 1780, and Seek No Further from Westfield, Massachusetts. In addition the Wethersfield orchard has Seckel and Bartlett pears, peaches, and cherries.

Fruit trees came almost with the first Pilgrims and each small farm had its orchard. A Mr. William Blaxton had an orchard at the foot of Beacon Hill in Boston as early as 1625 when he first came to Massachusetts. Ten years later, when he moved to Rhode Island, he grew Blaxton's yellow sweeting apple which was rich and delicious.

In 1633 the Dutch started the first Connecticut orchards in Hartford when they built a fortified trading

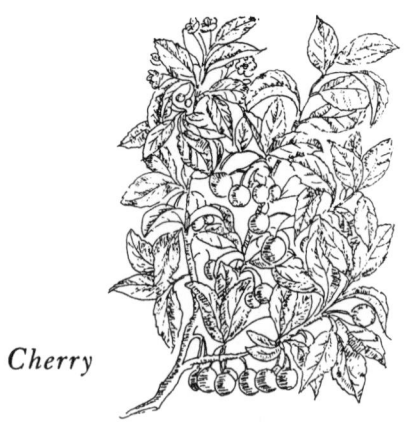

Cherry

post there. In 1641 George Fenwick of Saybrook, Connecticut, wrote, "I am prettie well storred with cherry and peach and did hope I had a good nursery of apples but the wormes have in a manor destroyed them all as they came up." An early nurseryman in Connecticut was Henry Wolcott, who in 1648 filled 32 orders for apples, pears, and quinces. He advertised Belle et Bonne and several pippins. Apples were most popular for cider. In a town of 200 families near Boston it was reported that 10,000 barrels of cider were made. People sometimes exchanged trees, as many as 500, for land. Most trees were grown from seed and, after five or six years, set in a pasture. Weak ones were weeded out and all were pruned high to permit the browsing of sheep.

In 1724 *Philosophical Transactions* said, "Our apples are without doubt as good as those of England, and much fairer to look to, and so are the pears. Our peaches do rather excell those of England."

In 1736 a Boston gentleman, Thomas Hancock, wrote an order for trees to James Glin, Stepney, England, in which he asked for dwarf fruit trees and espaliers. Alas, in 1737 he wrote back that half of the trees and all the seeds he had received were dead. A Boston newsletter of 1772 speaks of grafted fruit trees with a choice of three or four hundred sorts including "pares and plumbs." Westfield Seek No Further was the most popular apple along the Connecticut River from 1750 on.

Roses

Rosa Alba

So sweet a kiss the golden sun gives not
To those fresh morning drops upon the rose.

SHAKESPEARE, *Love's Labour's Lost*

Sixty references extoll the beauties of the rose in
Shakespeare's works. Rosa alba blooms in June with
double white flowers tinged with pink and is the source
for attar of roses. It is of unknown origin coming to
England from China through Persia, India, and Syria
to the Greek and Roman states. From the Romans
came the custom of crowning brides with roses and the
use of garlands of roses by noblemen as a preventive
of drunkenness. At important Roman dinners, if a rose
were hung over the table, it signified that the conversa-
tion was confidential; hence the term *sub rosa*. On their
conquering way across Europe, the Romans took the
rose to France, founding that country's most lucrative
perfume industry, then on to England where it was en-
shrined as the national emblem. Undoubtedly wild roses
had preceded their arrival. An Anglo-Saxon herbal of
the eleventh century speaks of a conserve of rose petals
"taken in the morning and fasting at night, it strength-
eneth the hearte and taketh away the shakings and
tremblings thereof." Later came England's War of
the Roses followed by a new Tudor rose with both red
and white blooms symbolizing unity.

3

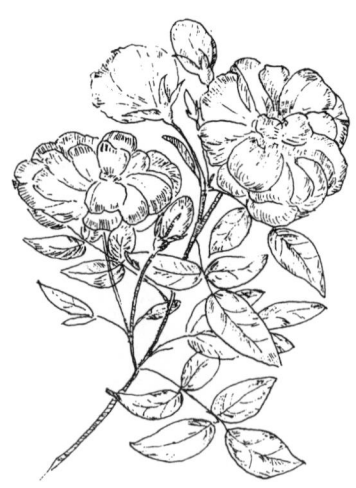

Rosa Mundi

Apart from its beauty, the rose has long been put to medicinal uses. Hippocrates included it among his "simples" and it is still used as a confection. An infusion of honey and red roses was used as a curative in the treatment of sore throat. The making of rose water, the distillation of rose extracts, the use of hips very strong in vitamin C for jellies and tarts, the history of the famous attar of roses, are each fascinating studies in themselves.

In Colonial times the Rosa alba, together with others, was brought from England to Plymouth where it is now known as the Plymouth rose. As in England, wild roses had long preceded the colonists as is proved by pre-Indian rose fossils found in Colorado; but the fine, imported English roses were always the featured plant in early gardens. John Josselyn wrote, "English roses do very pleasantly."

This scientifically-minded author published two little books in London which offer a wealth of information about Colonial plants in the seventeenth century. One is *New England Rarities Discovered,* 1672; the other is *Account of Two Voyages to New England;* 1673, reprinted 1675. He had come here to visit a brother in 1630 and again in 1663, remaining that second time for eight years. Careful notes in his diaries record what he found growing here. These books were reprinted in Boston in 1865 and are available in a number of libraries.

Bee Balm

Monarda didyma
perennial to 3 feet

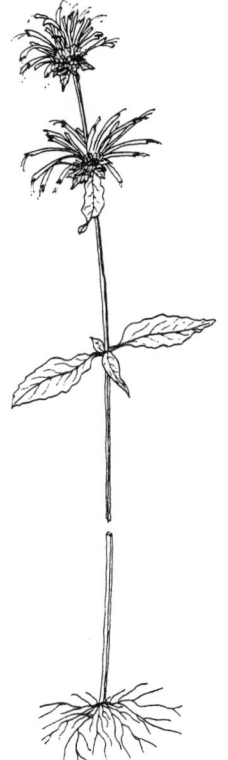

Speak not, whisper not
Here bloweth thyme and bergamot
Softly on thee every hour
Secret herbs their spices shower.

WALTER DE LA MARE,
The Sunken Garden

"When bees stray, they find their way home by it,"
wrote Pliny, the ancient Roman naturalist. Beekeepers
still make a plantation near their hives for the abundant
nectar stored in the blossoms. Peter Kalm, a Swedish
scientist and a traveler in North America, in 1748
wrote of the rivalry between humming birds for the
"monarda with crimson flowers." The blossoms have
a pungent lemon scent and the plant shows its kinship
to the mints in sending out spreading stolens. Jane
Colden, the eighteenth-century botanist, named it red
mint. It was also called bergamot, Oswego tea, or Indian plume and was much used in its native form by the
Indians. Colonists brewed a black tea for relief of colic,
fever, or colds and the oil was used for soap or perfume.
Surely they enjoyed it for garden color in the shady
border as we still do.

5

Betony

Stachys officinalis or Betonica
perennial to 3 feet

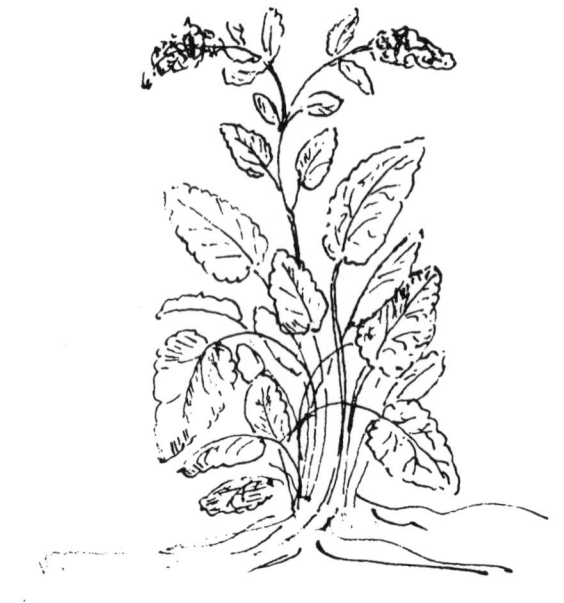

*Eat Betony or the powder therefor and you
cannot be drunken that day*

RYCHARDE BANKES, *Herball*

This is a "simple" well known to early settlers. History of its healing virtues for any and all complaints has come down to us from the ancient Greeks. An old Italian saying puts it, "Sell your coat and eat betony." The great scholar Erasmus believed the then-current superstition that betony was a charm against evil, prevented fearful visions, and drove away devils and despair. Bankes' *Herball* adds, "that if it be stamped and laid to a wound in the head that is smitten with a stroke, it shall heal the wound fair. Or take betony and stamp with water or with wine and drink it ten days, and it shall destroy any web (cataract) in the eye." It had a myriad of other medieval uses.

Bloodroot

Sanguinaria canadensis
perennial to 8 inches

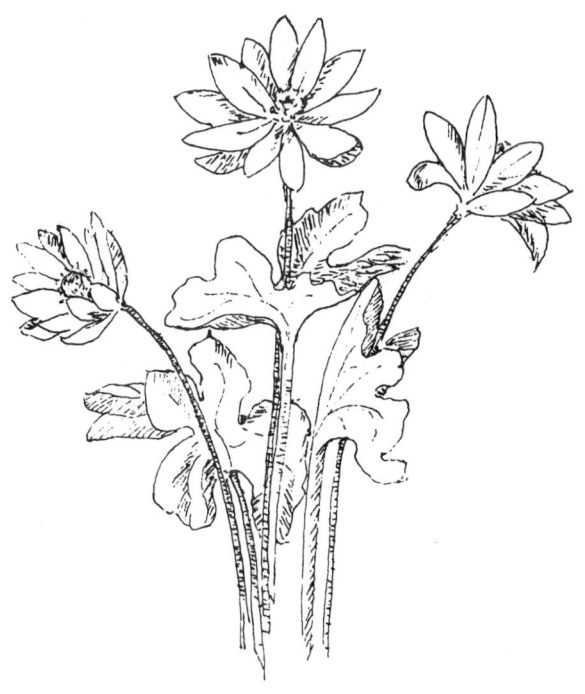

This little wildflower thrives in the forests of eastern North America in rich woods soil. It is also called red root or Indian plant and *sanguinaria* refers to its blood-like juice. Its red root sends up a red sap which the Indians used as a dye. Colonists welcomed this native addition for their dye pots which hung constantly in their kitchens. They also used other native plants for dyes: goldenrod for yellowish tans or old gold, dock for dark yellow, bayberry for gray-green, fiddleheads of fern or lichens for yellowish green, blackberry for light gray. Indigo was purchased for blue color in cakes or powder ready to use. A blue dye pot was said to receive as much service as a tea pot.

7

Indigo was imported readily from the Indies and itinerant peddlers made their rounds once or twice a year selling it at $2.00 a cake. It had largely supplanted the Saxon woad plant on which England had depended for blue until, by the seventeenth century, indigo from the East largely took its place. Woad had been a disagreeable plant exhausting the soil and bearing a very unpleasant odor when fermenting to make the dye. Queen Elizabeth I issued an edict that no woad should be grown within eight miles of any of her palaces because of the odor. It seems unlikely that the colonists would have cleared land for woad but they did send for seed since it was the native dye plant with which they were familiar. They must have been delighted to find bloodroot for red dye growing abundantly here, but we can be sure that early dyeing experiments with native materials were carried on by trial and error with many a disappointment. The whole subject of dyeing could be a book in itself. Currently, a group in Rhode Island has reproduced forty excellent dyes from native materials.

Dyeing in different utensils such as iron, copper, or tin produced quite different tones of the same basic color.

Candytuft

Iberis amara
annual to 1 foot

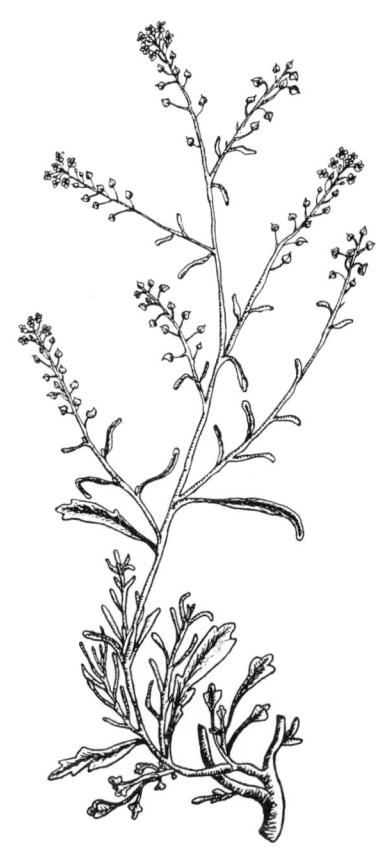

*The fairer and larger your allies or walks be,
the more grace your garden should have, the
less harm the herbes and flowers shall receive,
and the better shall your weeders cleanse both
the bed and the allies.*

JOHN PARKINSON

The snowy edging of candytuft makes fairer still such beds. It was grown for garden bloom but *A Curious Herbal* by Elizabeth Blackwell says, "The leaves and roots are commended by the ancient for Scrabia, being beaten into a cataplasm with hogs lard and applied to the part affected, and kept on four hours to a man, two hours to a woman and the place afterwards washed with wine and oil."

9

Carnation
Clove Pink

Dianthus caryophyllus
perennial to 2 feet

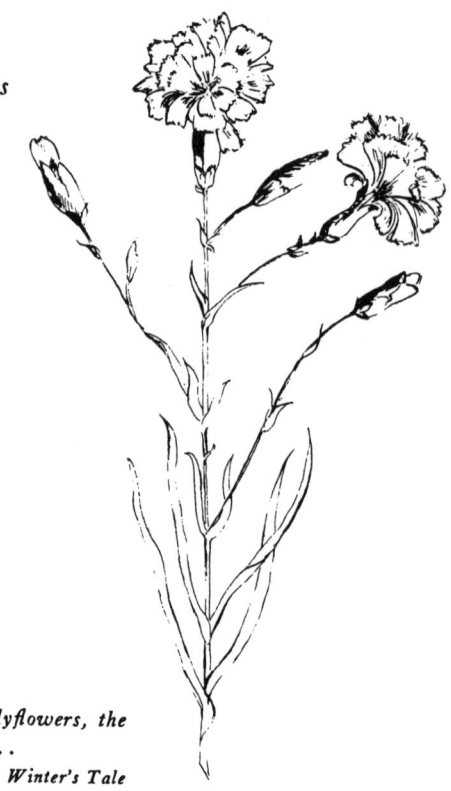

*Carnations and streaked gillyflowers, the
fairest flowers of the season . . .*
SHAKESPEARE, *A Winter's Tale*

Parkinson goes on to say that it is good for disorders of
the head and the best form is in a syrup made by pour-
ing 5 pints of boiling water upon 3 pounds of the
flowers, let stand for 12 hours and strain into 2 pounds
of sugar per pint. Gerard adds that "the conserve made
of the flowers . . . is exceedingly cordiall and wonder-
fully above measure doth comfort the heart, being
eaten now and then." Here it was grown more for
garden bloom but no doubt some early housewives
made the conserve for diseases of the head and heart.

*The clove gilloflower is most used in physiche
. . . and is accounted to be very cordiall*

JOHN PARKINSON

Catnip

Nepeta cataria
perennial to 3 feet

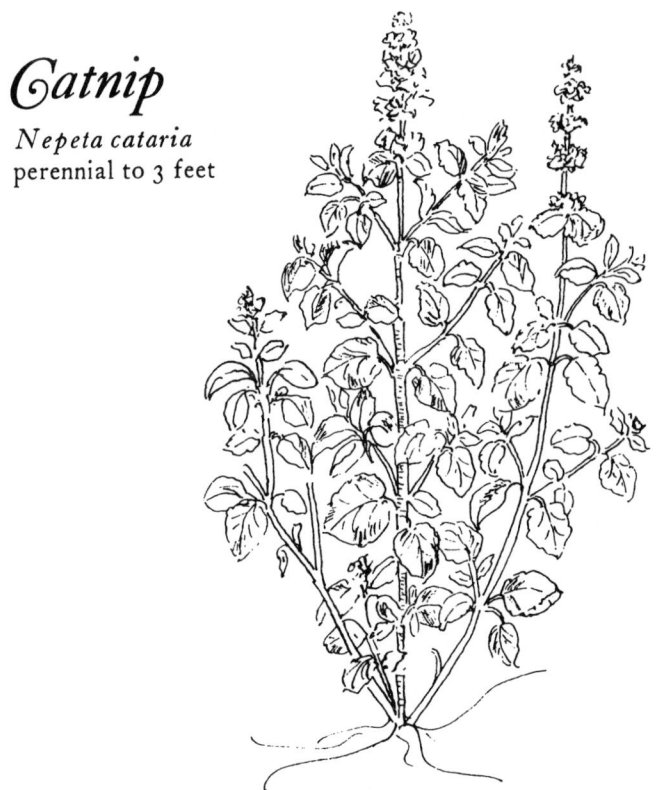

This is an old sweet herb widely naturalized in North America and much beloved by cats. In England it is called "Cat's Fancy." All who love cats have given them catnip in which to roll and seen the singular intoxication it brings. They become truly wild creatures, miniature tigers. Young plants are decorative in the garden but later become straggly in their full growth. Colonists made aromatic catnip tea from dried or fresh leaves, a handful to the cup. After steeping it for ten minutes, they strained it and flavored it with honey. In France this herb tea was served guests before retiring to help digestion, more effective perhaps than to-day's synthetic doses and pills. It is often sown on waste lands for bee forage.

There grows no herb of help to heal a coward heart.
SWINBURNE, *Bothwell*

Chamomile

Anthemis nobilis
perennial to 1 foot

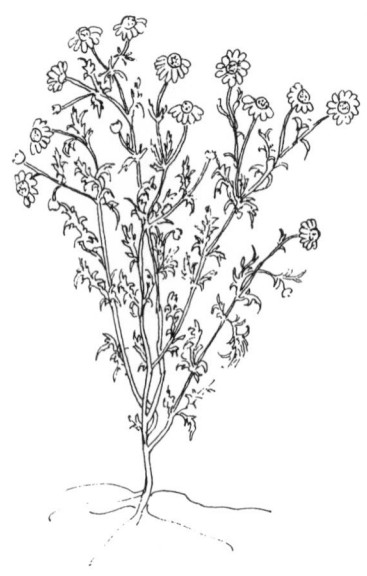

*Though the Camomile the more it is trodden
on the faster it grows, yet youth the more it is
wasted the sooner it wears.*

SHAKESPEARE, *Henry IV*

Chamomile is characterized by its sweet scent, rather like apples. The specific name *nobilis* indicates its many healing virtues. It grows profusely on the cliffs and downs of Cornwall making a close, springy, fragrant carpet. Treading on it spreads the seeds. From ancient times until today chamomile has been one of the most frequently used herbs for producing sedative effects: to quiet babies, as tea for nightcaps, and as a poultice for all sorts of aches and pains. Culpepper says, "The flowers boiled are good to wash the head and comfort both it and the brain." It was considered good for all kinds of digestive troubles and if drunken with wine will break the stone. Colonists could easily bring seeds and would have relied heavily upon this "noble" plant.

Here is a recipe for an herb bath to be taken for edgy nerves: flowers of chamomile, leaves of peppermint, sage, rosemary, and thyme all dried first and then sewed up in a cheesecloth bag to be dropped into the bath.

Chives

Allium schoenoprasum
perennial to 1 foot

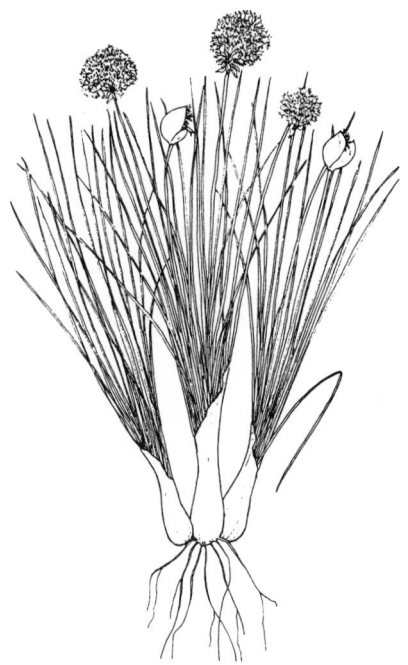

*He causeth grass to grow for the cattle
and herb for the service of man.*

Psalm 104

Chives belong with onions and garlic bulbs to the lily family. The original plants grew wild in North America, Europe, and Asia. It was then an indispensable seasoning as it is now. It was known to the Chinese as early as 3000 B.C. and was used all over Asia and northern Europe before the Christian era. Then it became a basic plant in monastery gardens and kitchens for seasoning soups, eggs, cheeses, and salads. The tiny bulbs were sometimes pulled and pickled. In addition to its culinary uses it was decorative with its small clover-shaped blossoms. It made an excellent edging for garden beds.

13

Crown Imperial

Fritillaria imperialis
bulb to 4 feet

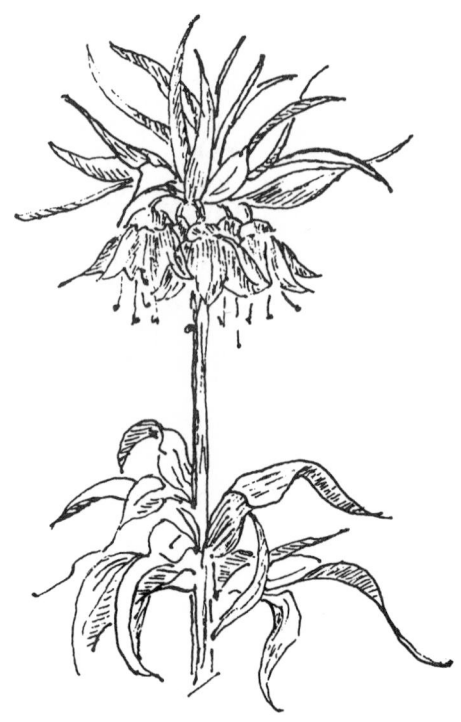

*The Crown Imperial for his stately beautifulness
deserveth the first place in this our garden of delight.*

JOHN PARKINSON

A native of Kashmir, this lily came via Constantinople
and Vienna to England. Only one other lily, the pure
white candidum, was more popular.

The botanical name is derived from *fritillus* or
chessboard alluding to the clustered coloring of the
flowers which are pendent and bell-shaped. An old
world favorite of easy culture, persisting for years, it
was consequently a dependable plant for dramatic
garden bloom.

Daffodil

Narcissus
bulb to 1½ feet

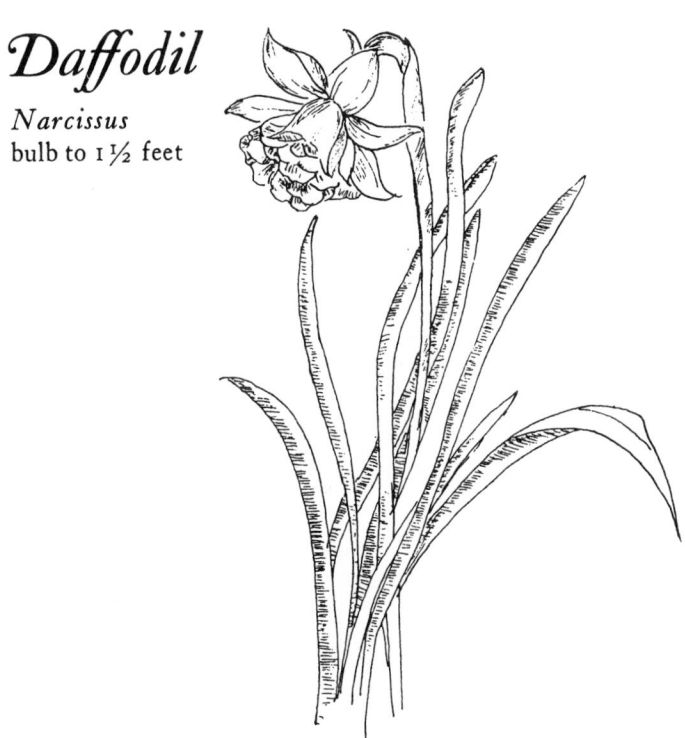

*Daffodils that come before the swallow dares
And take the winds of March with beauty.*

SHAKESPEARE, *A Winter's Tale*

The name may come from the old English *affodyle,*
that which comes early. Narcissus is from the well-
known myth of that name about the beautiful youth
who spurned the love of Echo. He was punished by
Nemesis who made him so fond of his own reflection
that eventually he became a flower.

Culpepper states that the roots, when bruised and
boiled with parched barley meal, healed fresh wounds.
If mixed with honey they strengthened sprains and relieved old aches in joints. Our colonists, no doubt, grew
them mainly for garden bloom to delight the eye at the
end of a long winter season.

In Wales they say that if you find the first bloom of
the season you will have more gold than silver that
year.

Day Lily

Hemerocallis flava
perennial to 3 feet

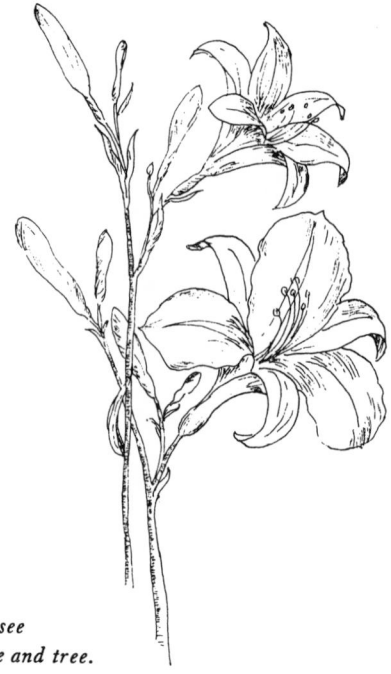

Get up sweet-slug-a-bed, to see
The dew despangling Herbe and tree.

ROBERT HERRICK
Corinna's going a Maying

Hemera means day in Greek and *kallos* means beauty, hence the botanical name, with *flava* added for bright yellow. The Greeks knew this garden favorite as a flower, beautiful for a day, each blossom shrivelling at day's end. It was grown for the uniform flowers above the mass of foliage and for the joy of its golden color to brighten the summer days.

It is interesting to note that most of the common garden flowers were Elizabethan or earlier in date. The favorite lemon day lily spread so gaily that it was often exiled from the front dooryard to the rear where a bank of lemon lilies in full flower brightened the day for many a colonial housewife.

Each Flower has wept, and bow'd toward the East
Above an houre since . . .

16

English Daisy

Bellis perennis
perennial 6–8 inches

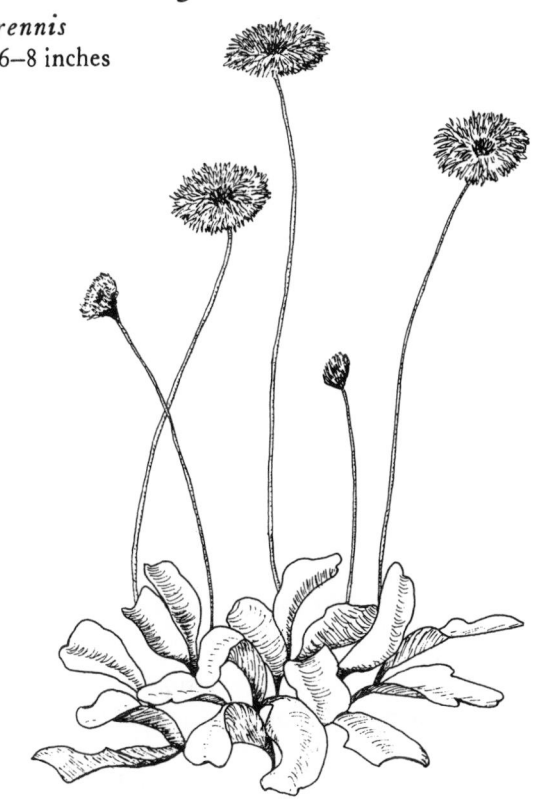

*The double daisies are planted in gardens;
the others grow wilde everywhere.*

JOHN GERARD

The word daisy comes from the Anglo-Saxon *daeges-eage*. Later Chaucer called it the "eye of the day." It was also called "bruisewort" because it was considered valuable for healing wounds, bruises, and boils. It was used in war as a salve for injured soldiers.

Daisies grow low like dandelions and originally had single white flowers tinged with red on slender stalks. They are members of the aster group of the composite family and were spread all over the world by Englishmen and most certainly came to Colonial New England.

Feverfew

Chrysanthemum parthenium
perennial to 2 feet

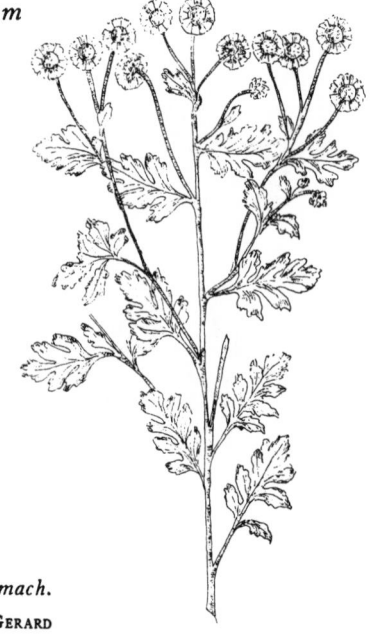

Its virtue is to comfort a man's stomach.

JOHN GERARD

Feverfew is a humble relation of the many-colored chrysanthemums. Dioscorides teaches that it was profitably applied to all hot inflammations and swellings. If dried and made into powder and mixed with honey or sweet wine, it alleviated vertigo, and was good for "such as be melancholike, sad, pensier, and without speech." It was also used for ague, as an antispasmodic in hysteria, and in Roman times for erysipelas and warts.

According to John Hill (1756), "The virtues of feverfew are very great. It is an excellent obstruent. It promotes the menses, and cures those hysterick complaints which rise from their obstruction. It also destroys worms."

Bees dislike it so much that a handful of the flower heads carried in a pocket will keep them at a distance. Consequently it must have been grown at a distance from the beehives which were such an important feature on Colonial properties.

Forget-Me-Not

Myosotis arvensis
biennial to 1 ½ feet

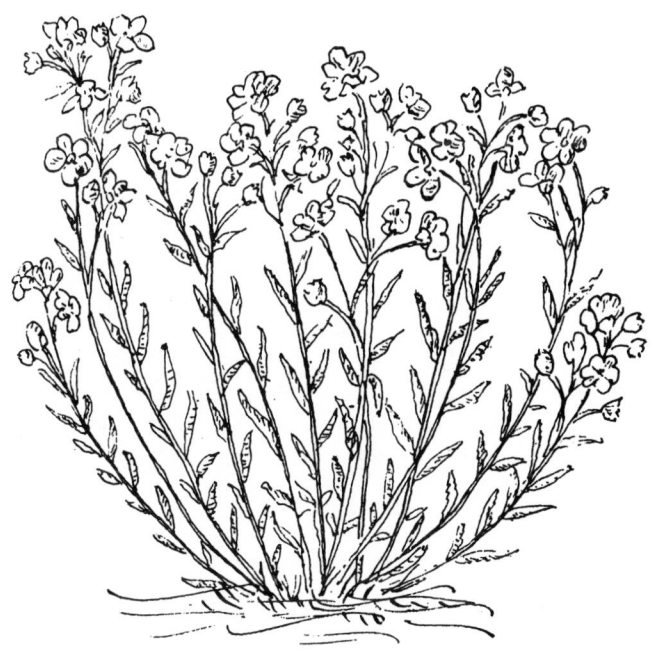

*It is said to be an astringent, but its virtues are
not certainly known.*

JOHN HILL, 1756

The beautiful blue and white color and low growth
makes the forget-me-nots very attractive as bedding
plants, especially as a carpet under tulips or other bulbs.
It is sometimes called mouse ear because of the shape of
the leaves. At one time it was customary to give forget-
me-nots to anyone starting on a journey on February
29. Later they were exchanged among friends on that
day. The colonists grew them for the delightful spring
bloom. The true forget-me-not is the symbol of faith-
fulness.

Foxglove

Digitalis purpurea
biennial to 4 feet

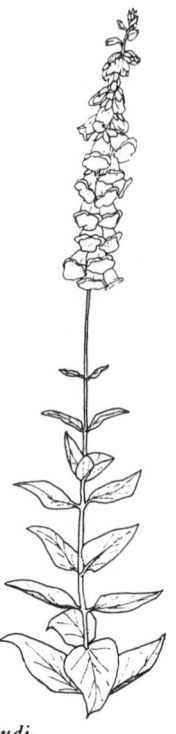

Foxgloves are not used in Physike by any judicious man that I know, . . . yet some Italians used it as a wound herb.

JOHN PARKINSON

This plant was also called fairy glove, finger flower, and lady's thimble. It was a native of England and a very popular garden plant before its medicinal use for heart ailments was first developed in 1785 by the British botanist, William Withering. It was used soon thereafter to lower the pulse rate in scarlet fever and tuberculosis. For the last hundred years, the drug has been grown all over the world and is the most valuable of all medicines for heart afflictions.

This important current medicinal use was developed after our Colonial period but here is what John Hill records of its virtues in 1756. "It is a plant possessed of very considerable virtues; but they are more known among the country people than in the shops. It is a powerful emetick, and, in a smaller dose, a very brisk purge; often it works both ways, and sometimes with a very hurtful violence but this is owing to ill management. Many excellent medicines, as they are found to be, in the hands of skilful persons, would fall under this censure if given in the same random manner. An ointment made of the leaves is recommended for cutaneous foulnesses, and in many places they make an ointment also of the flowers in May butter, which is greatly recommended in strumous cases. Many plants of less virtue are more celebrated; and there is none deserves better a fair trial."

Germander

Teucrium chamaedrys
perennial to 1 foot

Teucrium, a native of western Asia, is named for King Teucer, the legendary first king of Troy. *Chamaedrys* is from the Greek meaning "low" or "ground." Some species were used medicinally as far back as Hippocrates and Pliny. It was unknown to northern Europe until the sixteenth century. Dodoens, the Flemish herbalist, said it grew wild on the hills of his native Brabant. It was taken from there to England to fill the demand for small hedge plants. This was the period when elaborately patterned geometric borders and beds were very popular on the large estates of the aristocracy. Gerard grew it in his London garden and Francis Bacon enjoyed it in his winter garden. Box, rosemary, lavender, cotton, and hyssop were similarly used as hedge plants for the prevalent knot gardens. Germander was an ingredient in the eighteenth-century Duke of Portland's "Gout Powder" taken daily in wine. It came early to this country for its value as a small edging or hedge plant.

Grape Hyacinth

Muscari botryoides caeruleum
bulb to 1 foot

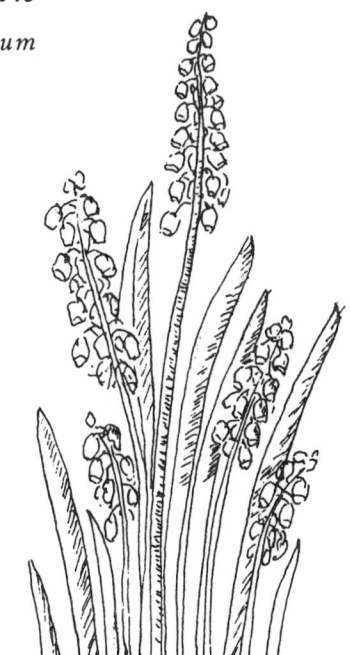

Take heed to thy bees, that are ready to swarm,
the loss thereof now is a Crown's worth of harm; . . .
Set hive on a plank, not too low by the ground
where herb with the flowers may compass it round;
And boards to defend it from north and north east,
from showers and rubish, from vermin and beast.

THOMAS TUSSER, *Mays Husbandry*

The Emperors Maximilian II and Rudolph II entrusted their garden of simples to the care of Clusius, or Charles de Cluse, a sixteenth-century botanist who also practiced medicine. In 1601 he listed *Muscari* as a plant from Constantinople. Actually it is native to the Mediterranean area. Grapelike flowers form clusters which attract bees to the early spring garden. We can picture the colonists' straw hives set out in their gardens surrounded by grape hyacinths and other bee plants.

Hollyhock

Althaea rosea
biennial 5 to 9 feet

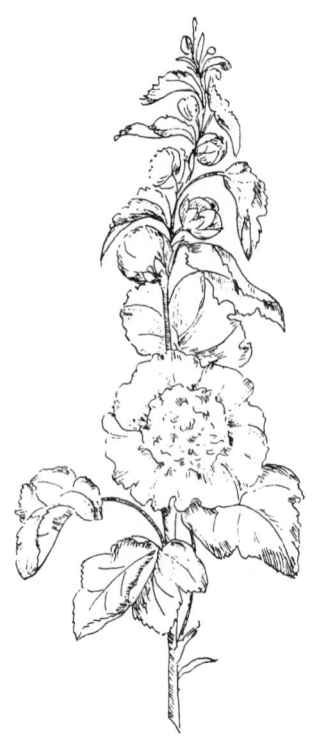

The word hollyhock is medieval English for Holy-Mallow, probably because it was brought from the Holy Land. *Althaea* means to cure. The plant was used by the Greeks in 200 B.C.

In 1735 John Custis of Williamsburg thanked Peter Collinson for his hollyhock seeds and they were advertised for sale in a Boston newspaper in 1760.

Early American colonists grew red, pink, and white single varieties. John Josselyn admired them in his *Two Voyages to New England 1638–1663.* The flowers were used for coloring purposes and immediately after picking were spread on trays in thin layers and placed in a current of warm air to dry.

The long thick root abounds in a mucilage differing little from gum arabic and has been used in cough medicines from ancient Egyptian times to the present. The large percentage of starch in the root, twenty-five percent, has made it popular for use in pastry and confectionery.

Houseleek

Sempervivum tectorum
rosettes 3- to 4-inch diameter

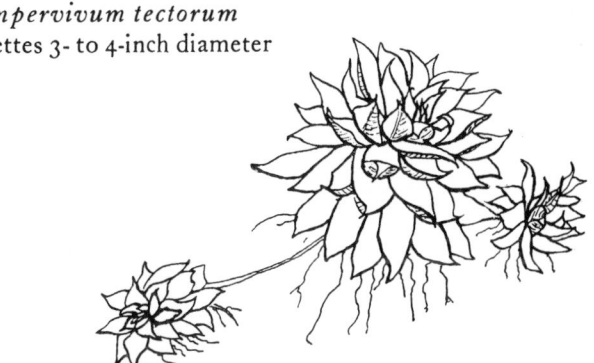

A cooling ointment may be made of the bruised leaves boiled in lard, which will answer all the purposes of the unguentum populneum.

JOHN HILL, M.D., 1756

Sometimes called hen-and-chickens, live forever, thunder plant, poor man's leaf. It is surprising that the familiar hen-and-chickens, a common plant, is a medieval herb with an interesting history. It is native to mountainous parts of Europe. Hippocrates boiled the thick leaves as a poultice for ulcers, a common ailment in ancient Greece. In Charlemagne's time it was used as an ointment throughout France and in a tenth-century manuscript it is called Semper-ins, or ever living, since it lives after uprooting. In 1562 a writer says "houseleke groweth in montagnes and hully places and some use to set it upon theyr houses." The belief grew that the plant growing on the roofs would keep away lightning and it follows that a damp thatch roof would not be an easy prey to fire. Today in England and Germany one still sees houses and barns topped with roofs vividly green with moss and houseleeks.

The leaves of the rosettes were an ever-ready source of strong astringent to stop the flow of blood from cuts and wounds, burns and scalds, St. Anthony's fire, and the shingles. Josselyn found them growing in Salem before 1672.

Hyssop

Hyssopus officinalis
perennial to 1 ½ feet

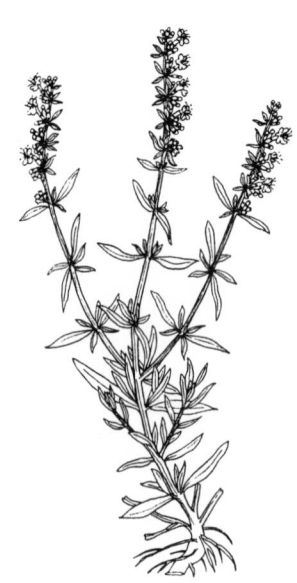

*Hyssop is the only fine sweete herb that I know
fittest to set or border a knot of herbs or flowers
because it will well abide and not grow too
woody or great nor be thinne of leaves in one
part when it is thicke in another so that it may
be kept with cutting as smooth and plaine as a
table.*

JOHN PARKINSON

Hence it was a fine hedge plant. The word immediately calls to mind the Crucifixion when Our Lord was handed a sponge soaked in vinegar dipped in hyssop.

The long, slender, dark green leaves have a mild mint odor. The spikes of closely set dark blue-purple flowers are valuable in attracting bees.

Thomas Tusser in his *Five Hundred Points of Good Husbandry,* 1597, lists it as a strewing herb to spread on walks and floors. Fragrant herbs were in great demand to strew on dirt, stone, or brick floors which were hard to sweep. Their refreshing perfume made the rooms sweet. In addition to its use for strewing, hyssop could be mixed with honey for cough syrup. A compress of the leaves steeped in hot water was excellent for removing black and blue spots.

Iris Pallida

Genus pogoniris
perennial 2–3 feet

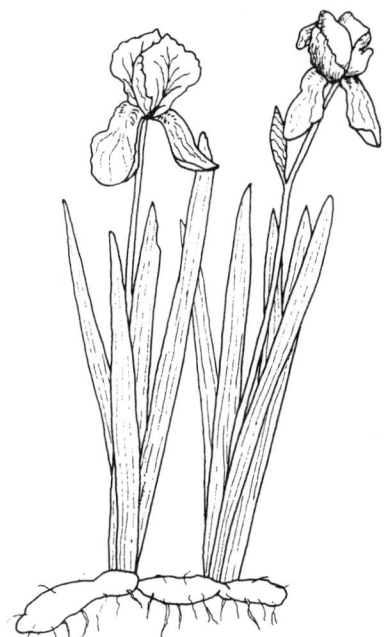

The iris is named for the Greek goddess of the rainbow because of its many colored flowers. *Pallida* is pale blue, and came to us from the South Tyrol. It is an important parent of the present bearded German Iris. It was the bearded iris which was grown extensively for the sweet smelling orris powder made from the roots after drying, pounding, and grating. The powder was a good snuff, also a cathartic and emetic.

However, the iris which became the flower of France in the time of Clovis (who used it on his shield) was yellow and not bearded. Louis VII adopted it for his heraldic emblem and it was contracted to "fleur-de-lys." Shakespeare in his *Henry VI* says "Cropped are the flower-de-luces in your arms; of England's coat one half is cut away."

In this country "Blew Flower-de-Luce" are mentioned by John Josselyn in his *New England Rarities.* Josselyn says, "It is excellent to produce Vomiting and for bruises of the Feet and Face." By the eighteenth century there are many references to the purple flag, iris versicolor, still well known in marshes and meadows. Like the fleur-de-lys of France it is beardless.

Jacobs-Ladder

Polemonium caeruleum
perennial to 2 feet

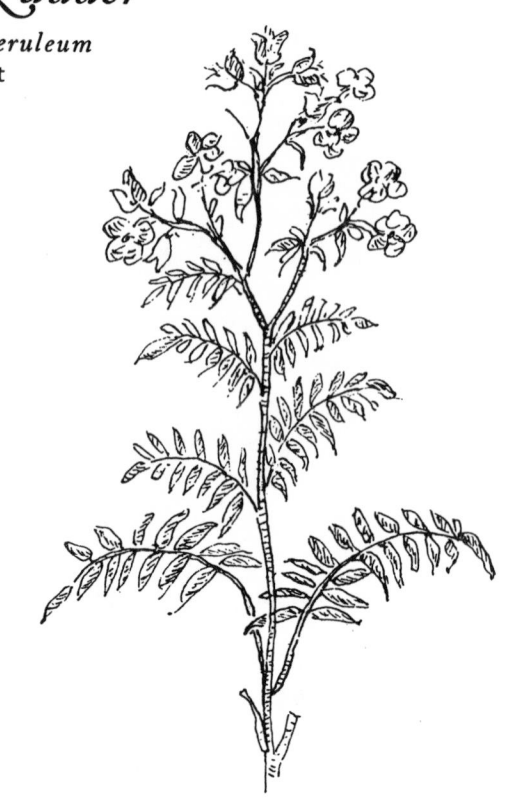

Talk to him of Jacob's Ladder and he would ask the number of the steps.

DOUGLAS W. JERROLD

This very hardy plant is the early Greek valerian. It thrives in sun or shade and multiples rapidly. The blue flowers are showy and the finely cut foliage resembles fern fronds. John Hill wrote in 1756, "Its virtues are unknown," meaning it did not have medicinal or culinary uses. What it did have was beauty for the colonists' spring gardens. It was worthy of widespread cultivation, but its botanical name had an unhappy connotation coming as it does from *polemos* meaning war in Greek. Pliny believed this plant led to war.

Johnny-Jump-Up

Viola tricolor
annual to 1 foot

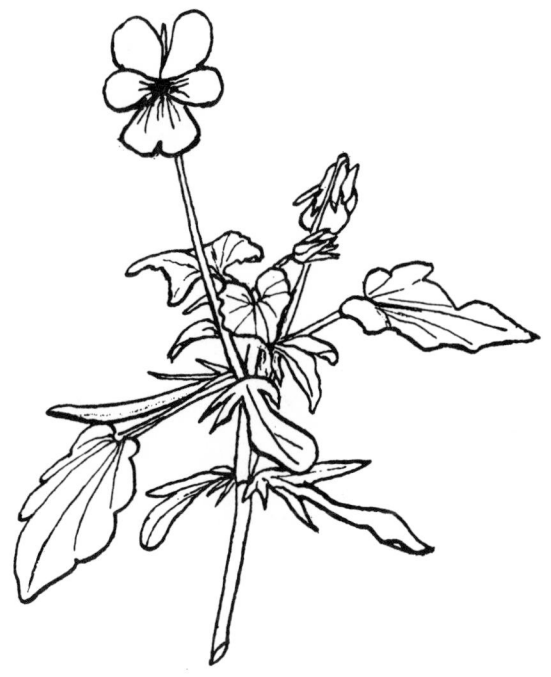

Pansies—that's for thought
SHAKESPEARE, *Hamlet*

The pansy of Shakespeare's time was the little Johnny-jump-up, also called heart's-ease, love-in-idleness, and herb trinity. "By reason of the beauty and braverie of their colors, they are very pleasing to the eye, for smell, they have little or none." The seed was advertised in Boston in 1760 and Jefferson reported planting it in his garden in 1767. The mature plants die but self-seed very freely so unless watched carefully Johnny-jump-ups can take over the whole garden. Colonists surely delighted in their persistent bloom and, perhaps, as their English ancestors had done, used the flower as a heart medicine.

Lady's-Bedstraw

Galium verum
perennial to 3 feet

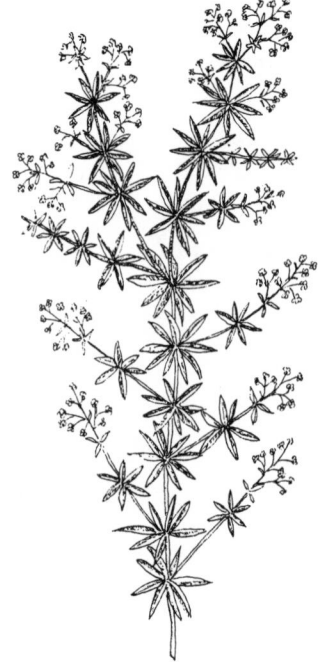

Arts perfect forms no moral need
And beauty is its own excuse;
But for the dull flowerless weed
Some healing virtue still must plead.

JOHN GREENLEAF WHITTIER

This plant is sometimes called Our-Lady's-Bedstraw because, according to a medieval legend, the plant was used during the nativity, and, as a reward, its white blossoms were changed to gold. The dried stems are soft and springy and do not crumble to dust. It was the softest available material for the couches of highborn ladies in the Middle Ages. Men could sleep on coarse straw!

The botanical name *Galium* comes from the Greek word *gala* meaning milk. Milk was curdled with galium as a substitute for rennet in the making of cheeses. This was a principal use, "Some commend a decoction of it for the gout and a bath made of it to refresh ye feet when tired with over walking." Another use that was of great value in Colonial times was as a dye. The chopped roots furnished a red color and the flowering tops produced a good yellow.

Lady's-Mantle

Alchemilla vulgare
perennial to 1 ½ feet

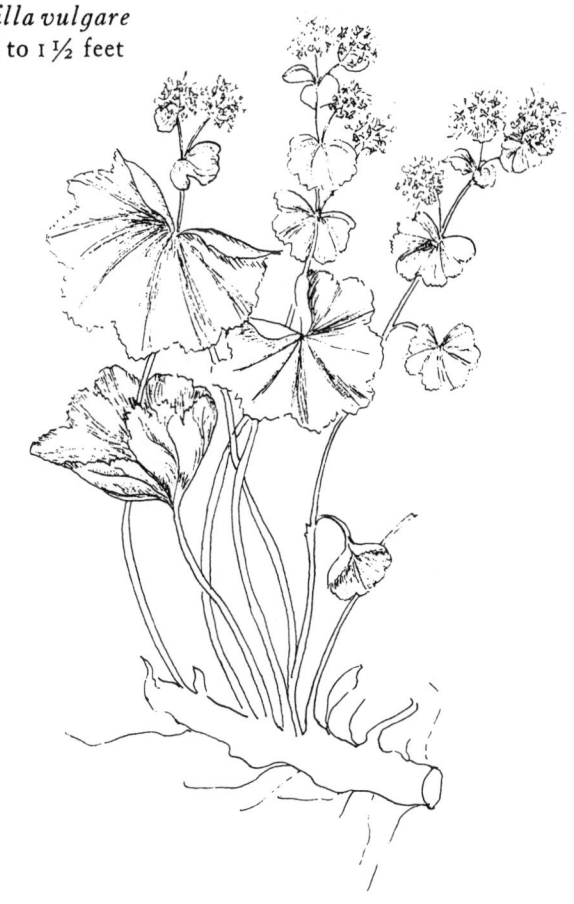

This low-growing almost evergreen member of the rose family has matlike foliage and greenish-yellow flowers. It is sometimes called lion's foot, bear's foot, and nine hooke. The leaves, which are pleated like a lady's mantle, hold dewdrops like jewels to sparkle in the early morning sunshine. The plant has considerable recommendation for herbal remedies being drying and binding "and of great force to stop inward bleeding." Applied outwardly the "leaves are accounted good for lank sagging breasts, to bring them to a greater firmness and smaller compass."

Lamb's-Ears

Stachys lanata
perennial to 1 ½ feet

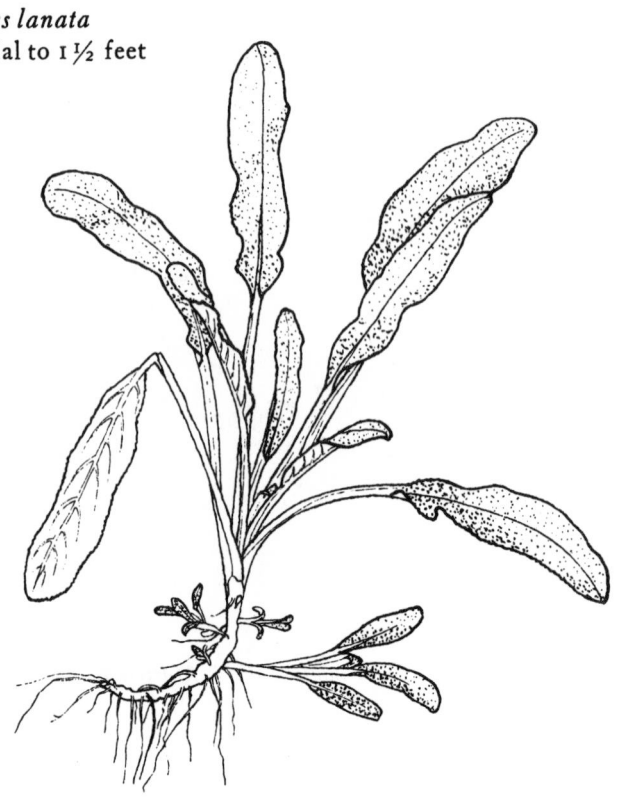

*Small herbs have grace, great
weeds do grow apace.*

SHAKESPEARE,
Richard III

This plant is also called lamb's-tongue from the shape
and texture of its leaves which are furry and grow close
to the ground. They make a splendid grey edging for
tall herbs in the garden. In late June the flower spikes
are showy and effective en masse. It was used mainly as
a bedding plant for it was not featured with the culinary or medicinal herbs in early records nor is it a
fragrant herb. The magenta flowers dry well for winter
bouquets.

Lavender

Lavandula officinalis
subshrub to 3 feet

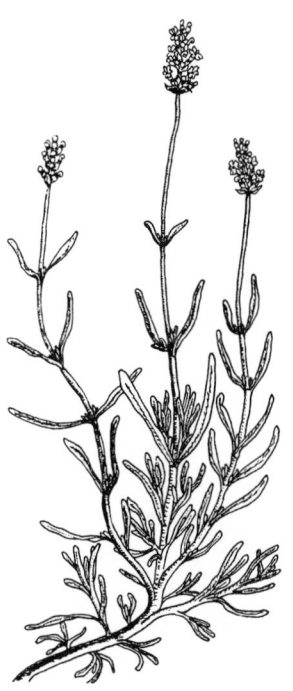

Here's flowers for you
Hot Lavender, Sweet mints, Savory, Marjoram,
. . . these are flowers of middle summer
and I think they are given to men of middle age.

SHAKESPEARE, *A Winter's Tale*

Lavender was a newcomer to England in Shakespeare's time. A native of southern France and the Canary Islands, it proved to be hardy and happy in England by the sixteenth century and became one of the most important plants in the herb garden. Its name stems from the Latin *lavo*, to wash, a reference to its use in lavender water. Its oil was considered effective against skin parasites and was used in soaps. Charles I of England granted a royal monopoly for making soap to a merchant named William of Yardly. Consequently lavender was grown for utility and needed in great quantity. It offered one of the few homegrown perfumes. Its fragrance warded off the evil smells of poor drainage and lack of sanitation and it was immensely popular.

For distilling the oil, the flowers were harvested in full bloom. Since the blossoms were beloved by bees, cutters in the lavender fields received "danger money" because of risk of stings. If sprigs were kept to dry they retained a permanent scent and were laid away with clothes and linens. Two teaspoons of the distilled water are said to have helped those who had lost their speech or voice. As a tea it was a headache remedy. Parkinson noted, "the dried flowers do comfort and dry up the moisture of a cold braine." Because of its many uses it was an essential plant for the Colonies.

Lavender Cotton

Santolina chamaecyparissus
subshrub to 2 feet

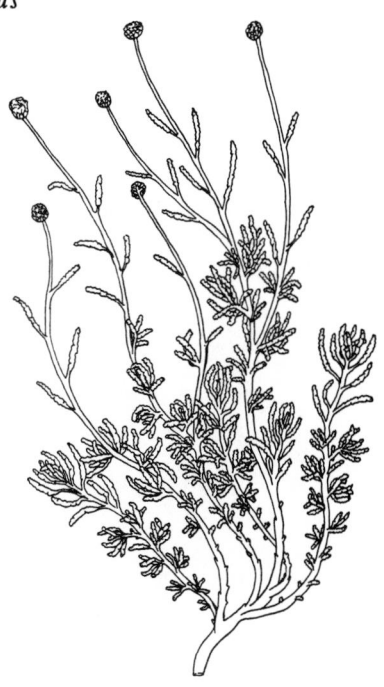

*The rarity and novelty of this herb, being
for the most part in gardens of great persons,
doth cause it to be of great regard.*

JOHN PARKINSON

This quotation refers to the extensive use of small
hedge plants for gardens so popular on the large estates
at the time. Lavender cotton was an excellent plant for
this purpose. It was imported from southern Europe
and its gray foliage offered a varied color note. It was
bushy at its base and could be clipped to form a compact
plant. The foliage was useful for its aromatic odor and
was laid away with woolens to repel moths. Some said
the leaves and flowers boiled in milk would destroy
worms and, infused in wine, it was considered a remedy
for jaundice. From early times it was popular in the
Colonies and was noted by John Josselyn in New England.

Lemon Balm

Melissa officinalis
perennial to 2 feet

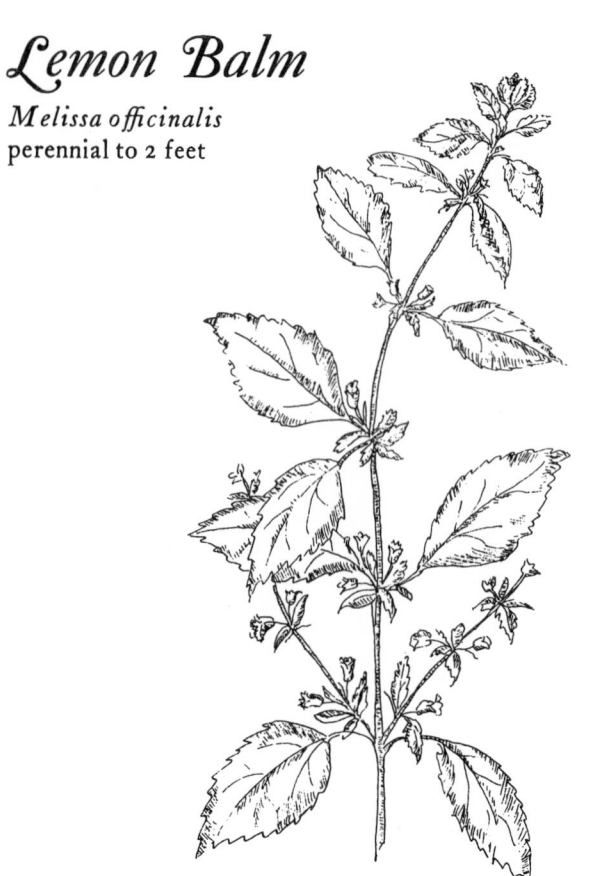

Lemon balm came from the mountainous regions of southern Europe. The name *melissa* is from the Greek for bee as it was a favorite bee plant. Virgil took great pride in his bees and grew balm especially for their use. It is a plant much beloved by the poets. Shakespeare refers to it in many of his works. It is mentioned in the *Bible* and in Homer's *Odyssey*.

Unlike some of the other herbs, balm was grown in flower gardens for its sweet odor as early as 1600 and was also included in bouquets. The foliage steeped in wine was drunk by the Greeks for fevers, and crushed leaves were used as a plaster for the stings of scorpions and the bites of mad dogs.

Commercial trading companies distributed the dry

herbage throughout much of Europe for use in medicine. Turner, in the 1664 edition of his *Herball*, refers to its power to drive away poisons arising from melancholy. Lemon balm was an ingredient of the famous Carmelite Water and was used along with honey as a potion to assure longevity. The oil was distilled and used in perfume and in furniture polish. Shakespeare says in *Merry Wives of Windsor*:

> *The several chairs of order*
> *Scour well with juice of Balm.*

When lemons were scarce, the dried leaves were added to jams and jellies. There was an ancient belief that bees would not leave a hive if there were plenty of balm nearby. As honey was an essential product for early kitchens this was another indispensable Colonial plant.

Lily of the Valley

Convallaria majalis
perennial to 8 inches

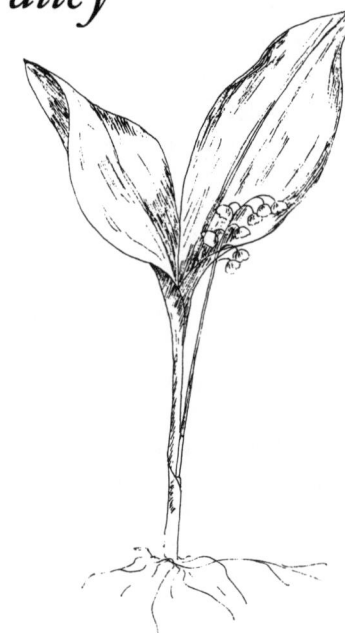

Convallaria is from the Latin word for valley; *majalis* is from Maiur or May since this fragrant plant blooms then. It is also called May lily and Our Lady's tears and is associated with the Virgin. It is a symbol of purity in religious painting.

The dried rhizome was a heart stimulant and was also used for epilepsy. The powdered root is still used to slow the pulse beat and as a diuretic for dropsy. The distilled water of the flowers was used for an eyewash for palsy and for apoplexy. Tea made from the flowers was considered excellent for all nervous complaints.

In addition to the important medicinal uses, lily of the valley was a valuable dye plant for our colonists. The leaves gathered in early spring made a fine pale greenish-yellow dye. When gathered in autumn they made a gold dye. A half pound of the flowers, soaked in a liter of wine for four weeks and then distilled, makes a liquor "more precious than gold. This wine smeared on the forehead and the back of the neck makes one to have good common sense."

Lovage

Levisticum officinalis
perennial 6 to 8 feet

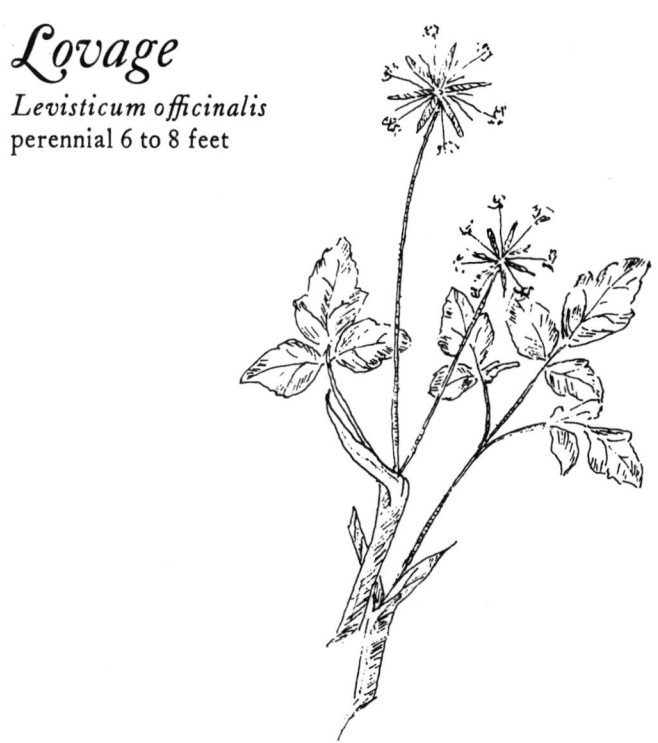

Lovage, an old-timer among the herbs dating from the eighth century, has been sadly neglected in modern times. It was used as a celery substitute by our forefathers, being easy to grow and having a strong celery flavor and aroma. If the seed heads are cut early, leaf growth is stimulated. If left to set seeds, birds, especially goldfinches, are attracted. The root used to be candied in sugar syrup and was called smallage at Shaker colonies where it was grown for sale. A lovage leaf will alleviate the pain from a bee sting if crushed and rubbed on the bite. The leaves are delicious in salads, soups, and stews and they were a source of oil for perfume. Culpepper says, "The distilled water helps the quinsy in the throat, if the throat and mouth be gargled with it, and it helps the pleurisy, if drank three or four times. It takes away the redness and dimness of the eyes if dropped into them; it removes spots and freckles from the face."

Lungwort

Pulmonaria officinalis
perennial to 10 inches

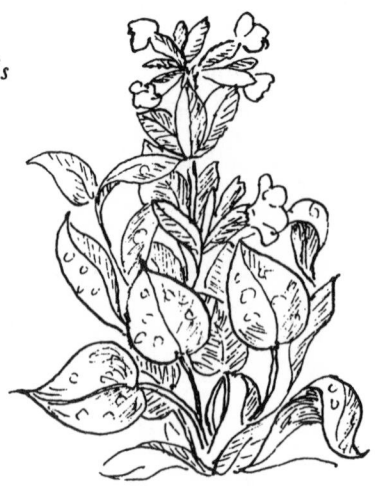

*It is much commended of some, to be singular good for
ulcered lungs—being boiled and drunk*

JOHN PARKINSON

Parkinson goes on to say that it grows naturally in the
woods in Germany but was found in England also by
John Goodier, "a good searcher and lover of plants."
There it was called "cowslip of Jerusalem" or "sage
of Jerusalem." It was sometimes known by the name
of "Joseph and Mary," its pink flowers being the emblem of Joseph and its blue flowers the emblem of the
Blessed Virgin. There is a legend that the Virgin's
tears fell on the leaves causing their white spots. The
name "soldier-and-his-wife" also referred to the red
and blue flowers. John Hill, 1756, says, "It is good in
the obstruction of the viscera and in the jaundice. The
leaves and fresh tops boiled in ale are a familiar medicine among the peasants of Germany." Here in the
Colonies, it was primarily enjoyed for its early spring
bloom.

> *When patients come to I*
> *I physicks, bleeds and sweats 'em*
> *Then—if they choose to die*
> *What's that to I—I let's 'em.*

AUTHOR UNKNOWN

40

Marjoram

Origanum vulgare
perennial to 2½ feet

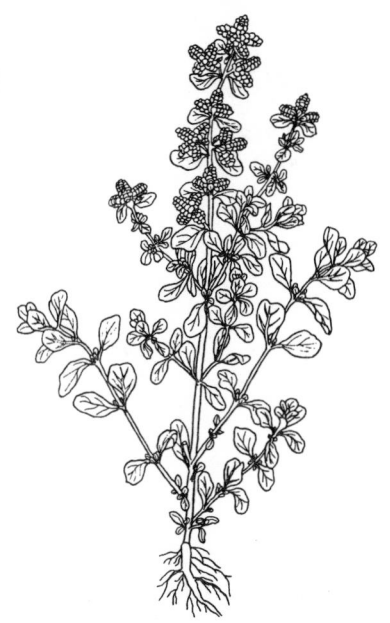

The leaves boiled in water and the decoction drunk easith such as are given to over much singing.

JOHN GERARD

Gerard called it "origanie" and marvelled that it remained green "all this long winter of 1597." The dark green foliage is a thick ground cover in the spring but later the flower stalks are tall and leafy too. *Origanum* means "joy of the mountains" and it is said that the flavor of goat's meat, served as a delicacy in Greece, comes from their foraging on oregano which grows on the mountain sides. In ancient times if marjoram grew on a tomb it was believed that the person buried there was happy.

It was introduced very early in Colonial gardens and escaped to grow wild along the roadsides. It was another dye plant for the housewife. The tops gave a purplish color to wool and a reddish-brown color to linen. Tea made from the leaves relieved spasms, colic, and indigestion. "It easith the tooth ache being chewed in the mouth. The leaves dried and mingled with honey put away black and blue marks."

Mint

Mentha piperita
perennial to 3 feet

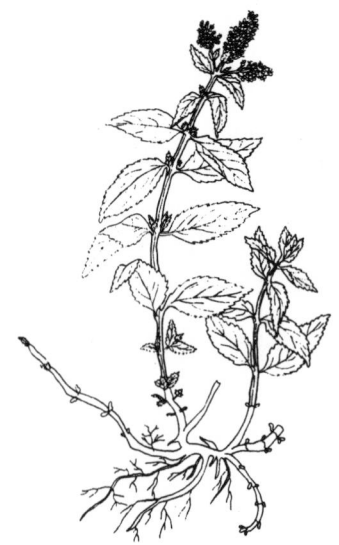

The smell of mint doth stir up the mind and the taste to a greedy desire of meat. Mint is marvelous wholesome for the stomach. It is good against watering eyes if poured into the ears with honeyed water.

PLINY

Menthe, daughter of Cocytus, was beloved by Pluto but because of the jealousy of Proserpina, she was changed into the humblest of plants to be trodden by all. Mint originated in Corsica and by the Middle Ages there were many varieties and many, many uses.

In colonial times mint was "A good posie for students to oft smell. It quickened the brain." Also, "It cooleth the tongue when added to beverages." It was brought here very early and was growing wild in New England by 1672 when John Josselyn spoke of seeing it. The leaves were used for flavoring drinks and food, the oil for perfume and medicines.

In Bolivia the people believe that anyone who finds mint in bloom on St. John's Day will have happiness forever.

Give peppermint for baby's gas
For older folks just use Sasafras.

AUTHOR UNKNOWN

Parsley

Petroselinum
biennial 10 to 15 inches

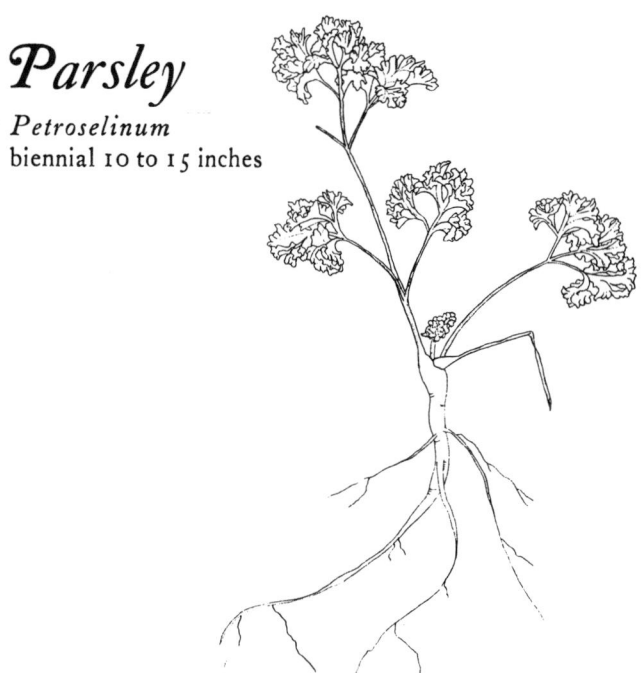

*It multiplieth greatly a man's blood. . . . It is
good for the side and the dropsy. It comfor-
teth the heart and the stomach.*

RYCHARDE BANKES, *Herball*

Parsley has been used since ancient times for soups, stews, herb omelettes, and all sorts of seasoning. Hercules is said to have selected parsley to form the first garland he wore. The name is from petros meaning rock as it grew on rocky soils in Greece. It is full of minerals, hence its value throughout the Middle Ages right up to the present time. In the pre-vitamin era of Colonial times it was especially appreciated and it is surely the most well known of all herbs.

The very slow germination of the seed gave rise to the old English rural saying that parsley seeds travel to the devil and back nine times before they sprout. "It is unlucky to transplant it and where it flourishes, the missus is master." It was brought to Newfoundland before 1620 by a British sea captain, John Mason. The Plymouth colonists grew it in their first gardens.

Peony

Paeonia officinalis
perennial to 3 feet

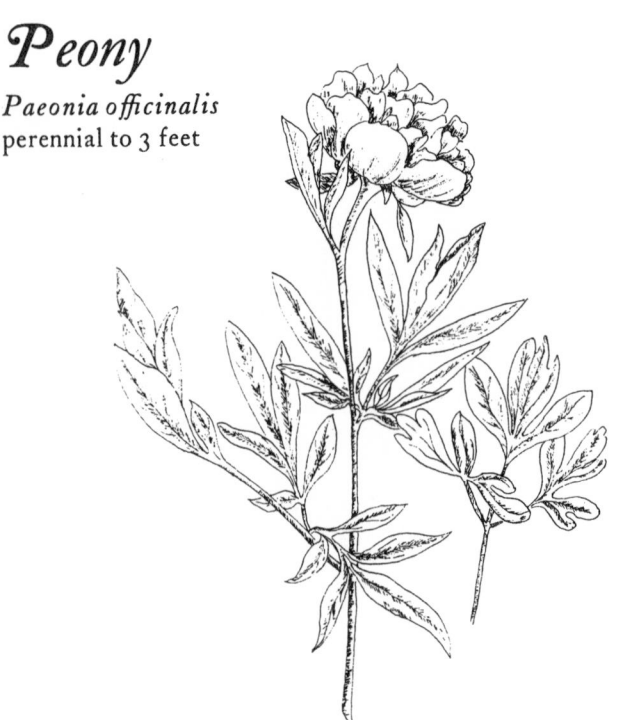

This erect herb growing from tuberous or thickened roots is named for a Greek god of healing, Paeon. Another legend is that the physician, Peon, used the roots to heel the wounds of Pluto. "This plant is accounted good for the Epilepsy, Apoplexy, and all kinds of nervous affections, both in young and old."

Tusser speaks of the peony as a physic herb. Beads made from dried roots were strung as a necklace to ward off convulsions. Some people carried dried seeds as a charm against evil. Colonists were particularly proud of the beautiful big flowers and, when possible, planted peonies in their front dooryards for the world to see and admire.

In Europe, in the Middle Ages, superstitious gardeners dug its roots by the light of the moon to avoid observation by woodpeckers. It was believed that if woodpeckers looked on anyone digging or planting peonies he would be struck by blindness.

Periwinkle

Vinca minor
trailing evergreen

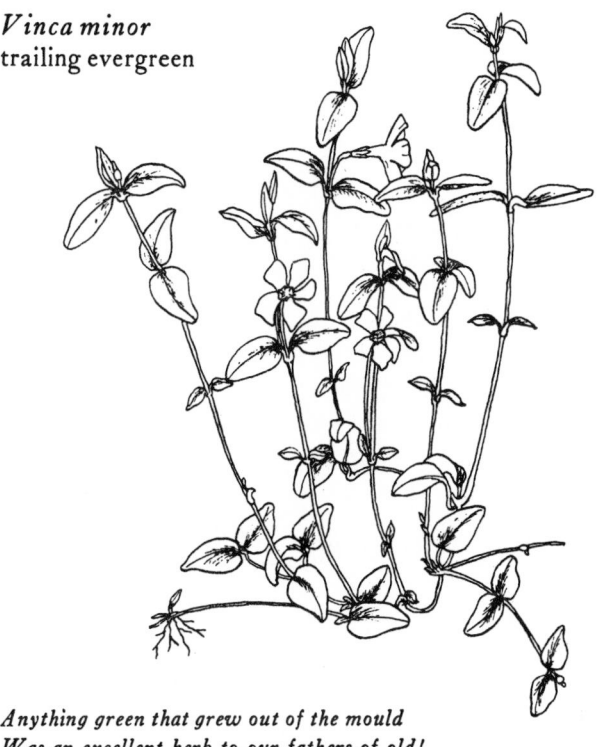

Anything green that grew out of the mould
Was an excellent herb to our fathers of old!
RUDYARD KIPLING

This low, sturdy, creeping plant has been grown in Britain for so many hundreds of years that it is considered native, but actually it came from the continent. Pliny mentions its cultivation in Rome in the first century and Chaucer refers to it.

The glossy green leaves all year round made it a popular ground cover in sun or shade and the unique blue flowers have a happy habit of blooming at almost any time of year, though most abundantly in the spring. Country people have long used it to make soothing ointments for the skin, and it is a tonic for intestinal troubles. In 1771 Jefferson included the plant in his plans for the garden at Monticello. It was a basic plant for all the Colonies.

Phlox

Phlox divaricata
perennial to 18 inches

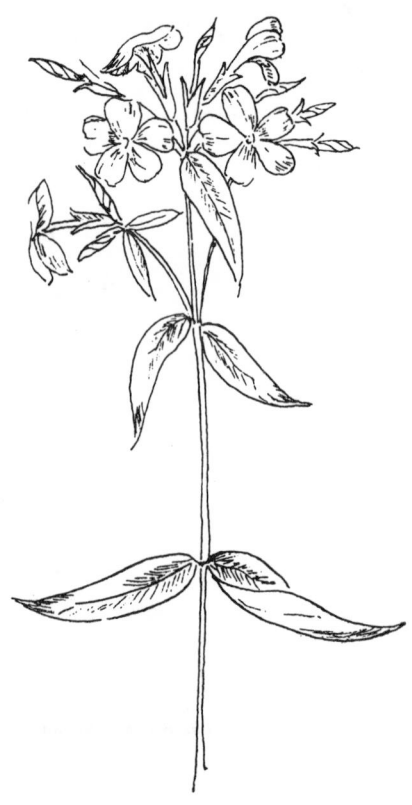

A blade of grass, a simple flower
Culled from the dewey lea
These, these, shall speak with touching power
Of change and health to thee.

FROM A SHAKER
HERB CATALOGUE

The name phlox is from the Greek word for flame, in allusion to the colors. *Divaricata* is sometimes called blue phlox or wild sweet William. It is a mass of fragrant blue-violet blossoms in May and is a charming adjunct to the bright tulip so cherished in Colonial gardens. The creeping stems root, increasing the size of the plant rapidly, and summer cuttings are made easily for new plants. This prolific, dependable flower was valuable for garden bloom. No references seem to be made to medicinal or culinary uses.

Pot Marigold

Calendula officinalis
annual to 2 feet

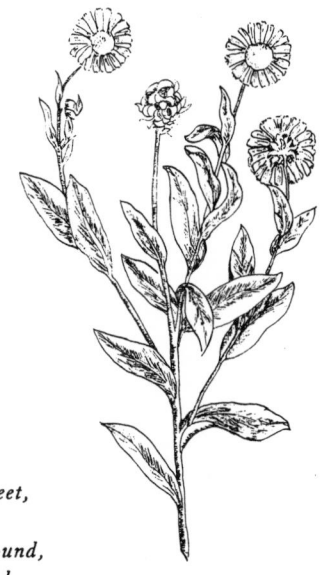

We walk'd abreast all up the street,
Into the market up the street:
Our hair with marigolds was wound,
Our bodices with love-knots laced,
Our merchandise with tansy bound.

WILLIAM BELL SCOTT
The Witches' Ballad

The marigold was mentioned by Josselyn in 1672 and it was brought to America by our first colonists. It was classed as an herb rather than a flower because of the yellow coloring matter which could be extracted. The "golds" were almost an invulnerable armor against witchcraft. Yellow flowers were protective because they reflected the sun.

Marigolds enjoyed a medicinal reputation in the Colonies with more basis in fact than many of the other old-time herbs. Tea made from it was good for fevers, measles, and jaundice. The juice of the petals relieved toothache. A conserve of the flowers aided the heart. The leaves flavored soups and salads.

In the First World War the marigold was used as a hemostatic. Physicians prescribed it in ointment form as a mild astringent for skin infections. In the Plymouth Colony it was also used for dying fabric, and it is still used to color and flavor cheese and margarine.

Primrose

Primula veris
perennial to 8 inches

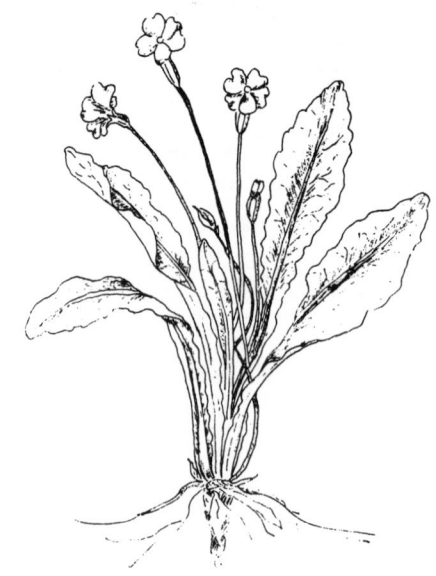

Now the bright morning star, days harbinger,
Comes dancing from the East, and leads with her
The flowering May, who from her green lap throws,
The yellow cowslip and the pale primrose.

JOHN MILTON, "On May Morning"

Primrose, loved by all English poets as well as by
Shakespeare, is also known by the more common name
of butter rose and English cowslip. It was native to
England, growing in dry meadows and pastures. The
soft yellow flowers resembling a bunch of golden keys
gave it the name of key flower and herb Peter. "Experi-
ence likewise, has showed that they are profitable both
for the Palsie and paines of the joynts . . . , which has
caused the names of Arthetica, Paralysis, Paralytica to
be given them," says John Parkinson.

It was useful in treating ordinary headache. The
whole plant had a mildly narcotic effect. The cure sug-
gested was one teaspoon of the flowers and leaves cut
small to one cup of boiling water: drink cold during the
day. A delicious wine was made from the flowers alone.
Leaves were used in salads, puddings, and tarts.
Flowers were candied or pickled and made into cowslip tea, syrup, or conserve. The syrup soothed nervous excitement. Juices from the flowers cleansed the
skin and took away wrinkles.

Rosemary

Rosmarinus officinalis
subshrub to 6 feet

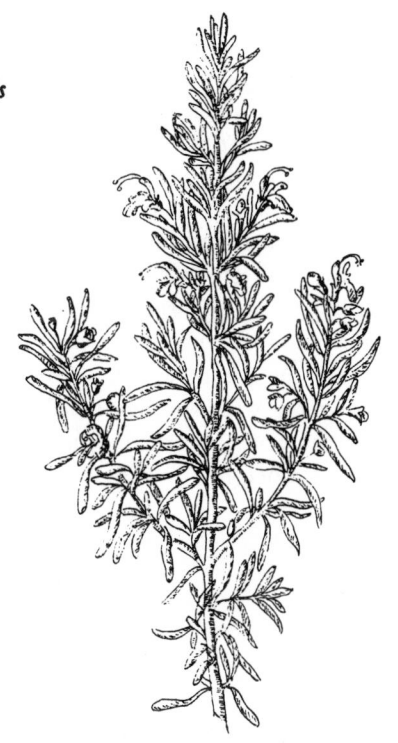

There's Rosemary, that's for remembrance;
Pray you love, remember.

SHAKESPEARE, *Hamlet*

The name is from the Latin word for sea dew because
the plant was found on the sea cliffs of southern France.
It has the smell of the sea and the tang of pines. It is a
native of southern Europe and is perennial in warmer
climates. Here it must be brought indoors in the winter.
The leaves are fragrant with touching but more so when
rubbed. When in full bloom, the plant is so fragrant
that baths were perfumed with it. Oil of rosemary is
made by distilling the leaves and tips. Eau de Cologne
cannot be made without it and it is used also in hair
and tooth washes. Its distinctive taste enhances breads
and boiled meats. Often a few chopped leaves were
added to wedding cakes or puddings. It was also a
strewing herb for floors.

Rosemary is best known as the emblem of remembrance and fidelity. Sprays of rosemary tied into the bride's bouquet signified happiness which never failed. A favorite valentine was a sprig of rosemary painted on a heart. At funerals a sprig was given each mourner to be dropped on the coffin.

There are two charming early legends, One tells of the Virgin Mary in her flight to Egypt with the Christ Child. She spread her cloak over a bush which happened to be the rosemary and ever after the flowers were tinged with blue, caught from the blue of the cloak. Another legend compares the growth of the rosemary with the height of the Saviour and declares that after 33 years the plant increases in breadth but. never in height.

Rue

Ruta graveolens
subshrub to 3 feet

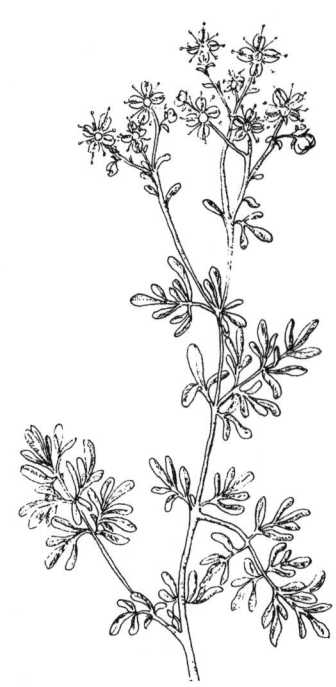

If your hound by hap should bite his master
with honey, rue, and onion make a plaster.

SIR JOHN HARRINGTON, 1608
The Englishman's Doctor

Rue was at its greatest popularity when the first colonists arrived in New England. Governor Winthrop grew it in his Boston Common garden.

No other herb except possibly rosemary has appeared as often in literature. Very early in history rue was symbolic of repentance. The word was derived from the old English *hreow* meaning to be sorry for. It became known as the "Herb of Grace" because it was used to sprinkle holy water in the churches. It was also an ingredient of charms worn to ward off evil influences. When witches in France took to the air on a broomstick they cried:

By yarrow and rue
And my red cap too
Hie—over to England.

The French used it to keep away moths, calling it *garde robe*. It had such a reputation as a disinfectant that in Elizabethan England it was strewn on the floors of the courts before prisoners were taken in so the justices would not catch "gaol fever." Pliny cites eighty-four remedies in which it was an ingredient and he said, "It is one of the most active of all medicinal plants."

Some said that it grew best if the plant had been stolen and that it thrived only where the mistress was master.

It was used to prevent nightmare. The seeds or leaves were pounded and mixed with vinegar until they became a mass. This was then added to old ale and strained for the patient. It was thought to be valuable in curing ailments of the eye and this led to the belief that it would give "second sight." When combined with sugar as a conserve, it was considered a remedy for epilepsy and hysterical complaints arising from the suppression of the menses. Rue was considered of value as an antidote to the bite of mad dogs and venomous creatures such as bees, salamanders, and serpents.

Sage

Salvia officinalis
subshrub to 3 feet

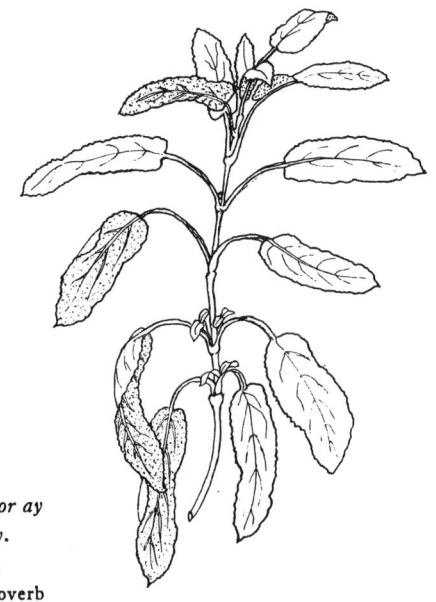

*He that would live for ay
must eat sage in May.*

JOHN RAY, 1678
Old English Proverb

Some old people attribute their longevity to sage tea in spring and autumn, sage sandwiches, and sage added to porridge. The plant grows wild along the northern shores of the Mediterranean. *Salvia* means to heal and *officinalis* means medicine. A conserve of the flowers will "warm and comfort the brain and nerves." The tea checks colds, fevers, and all sorts of ailments. For sauces and meat stuffing sage is almost as essential as salt and pepper. Gerard said, "It is singular good for the head and braine, quickeneth the senses and memory, strengthens the sinews, restoreth health to those that have the palsie." An old Arab proverb reads, "Why should a man die who has sage in his garden?" It is the herb of wisdom and immortality and has been valued by both East and West. There was a time when exchanges were made between the Dutch and Chinese of four pounds of tea for one pound of sage. The plants were so valuable that it was once the custom to plant rue near them to guard against toads. Pepys's *Diary* refers to a little churchyard in England with its graves covered with sage to mitigate grief. John Josselyn in his diaries noted it in New England.

Southernwood

Artemisia abrotanum
perennial to 4 feet

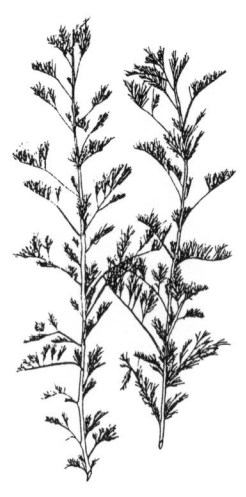

The garden border where I stood
Was sweet with pinks and Southerwood
JEAN INGELOW, *Reflections*

Here is a very hardy aromatic plant of many names: old man, lad's love, Saxon suthe-wurt, medieval sither wode. In Roman times Horace said, "None but a professional man dares prescribe Southernwood for a patient." The Greeks used it for cramps. *Bankes' Herball* in 1525 said, "The virtue of this herb is thus, that if they break the seed and drink it with water, it healeth men that have been bitten by any venomous beast." It was a favorite in old European monasteries and castle gardens. Young shoots were used in flavoring cakes and other foods. The French called it a *garde robe* and sprinkled the dried leaves in closets to keep moths away. Pennsylvania Germans used it in their pantries to keep away ants. Seeds and the dried leaves were given children to kill worms. The ashes of the dried herb mixed with oil were rubbed on the face to cause hair to grow, hence the name of lad's love. With bee balm and Bible leaf, southernwood sprigs made the posies tucked into many a Sunday dress to sniff during the long hours of church.

It was hung about courtrooms to avert jail fever and was used in kitchens to dispel cooking odors. A pinch on the open fire wafted a most pleasant fragrance through the house.

Star of Bethlehem

Ornithogalum umbellatum
bulb to 1 foot

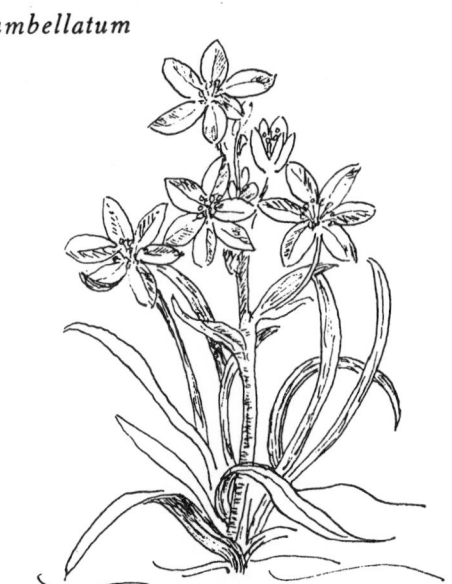

*The virtues of these plants are unknown, but
their beauty has given them a place in gardens.*

JOHN HILL, 1756

Though originating in the Mediterranean, the May-
blooming star of Bethlehem became widely naturalized
in eastern North America. The bulbs increase so
quickly they can become a nuisance in beds or borders
so they were mostly planted in wild gardens. They required no attention and their starlike white flowers were
a lovely carpet in woodsy areas. They must have sug-
gested the famous star of the nativity. They were also
called summer snowflake and sleepy Dick.

The botanical name is compounded of the Greek
ornies meaning bird and *gala* meaning milk. In the
Orient the bulbs were roasted for eating. That the
seeds were in demand in 1760 is proved by a Boston
newspaper seed list advertised on March 30 of that
year including star of Bethlehem with other popular
flowers.

Strawberry

Fragaria virginiana
perennial to 8 inches

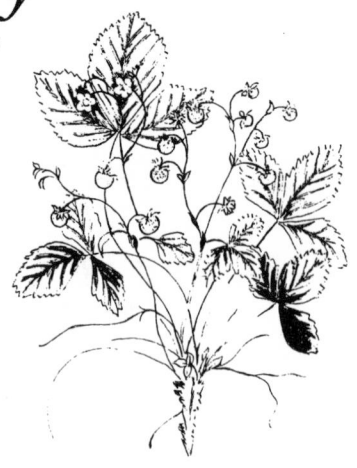

This is the common wild strawberry of eastern North America with small, very sweet fruit and rooting runners. The American variety has longer flowering stems and more elongated fruit than its European cousin. Tufted plants often grow thickly together offering a good supply of the delectable berries which must have been a particular treat in early times. The leaves were used in lotions and gargles for sore mouths and throats, or ulcered gums. Without good dentistry, they must have been in demand for the latter purpose. Some recommended them for jaundice and all kinds of fluxes. According to Elizabeth Blackwell "The fruit is accounted cordial and good for the hot bilious constitution." John Hill adds, "Also, it is good to destroy the web in a man's eyes. Also the juice of it meddled with honey and drunken, helpeth the milt."

> Wife, into thy garden, and set me a plot,
> With strawberry roots, of the best to be got;
> Such growing abroad, among thorns in the wood,
> Well chosen and picked, prove excellent good.
>
> TUSSER, *September's Husbandry*

This good advice to the English housewife would have been remembered in the Colonies where there was an abundance of luscious wild strawberries.

Sweet Cicely

Myrrhis odorata
perennial to 3 feet

Hard by, a cottage chimney smokes
From betwixt two aged oaks, where
Corydon and Thyrsis met are at
Their savoury dinner set of
Herbs and other country messes
Which the neat Phyllis dresses.

JOHN MILTON, *L'Allegro*

Myrrhis is from the Greek word for perfume. The ancient Greeks valued this plant for food and medicine. It is graceful and aromatic and could be used as a flavoring. The roots, divided in October or March, were eaten boiled like parsnips. Both the roots and the leaves were recommended for coughs and colic, and juice from the root was drunk "against the plague." It was known in Saxon times "being not uncommon as a salad." The large dark brown seeds were ground fine in the seventeenth century and used for polishing and perfuming oak floors and furniture. In addition it was a hardy decorative subject for the back of a garden border and was so used in Colonial days.

Sweet Woodruff

Asperula odorata
perennial to 8 inches

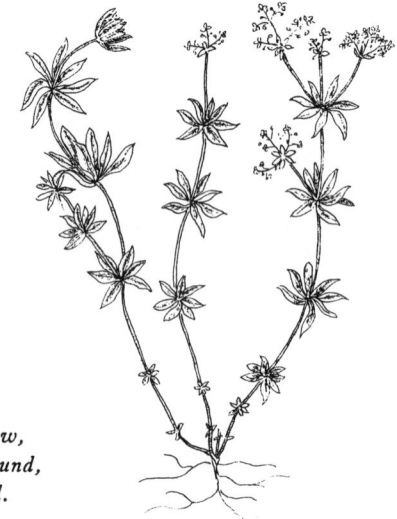

As aromatic plants bestow
No spicy fragrance while they grow,
But crushed or trodden to the ground,
Diffuse their balmy sweets around.

OLIVER GOLDSMITH,
"The Haunch of Venison"

Woodruff's chief virtue is its sweet odor making it one of the best of the strewing herbs. Rushes and meadow hay were adequate on floors for ordinary days, but for festivals, Sunday, weddings, and funerals other sweet-smelling herbs were added. They were grown for the purpose.

Its flowers look like tiny white stars. Gerard says, "The flowers grow at the top of the stemmes of a white colour and of very sweet smell, as is the rest of the herb, which being made into garlands or bundles and hanged up in the house in the heate of the day, doth very well attemper the aire, coole and make fresh the place, to the delight and comfort of such that are therein."

Saxon books of 1000 A.D. refer to "Wuderofe" as valuable in smelling salts for headaches but it was never an important medicinal or pot herb. It was a German custom to place sprigs in white wine to make "Maiwein," a custom still followed today. It was considered a tonic because it contains coumarin, a blood thinner.

Tansy

Tanacetum vulgare
perennial to 3 feet

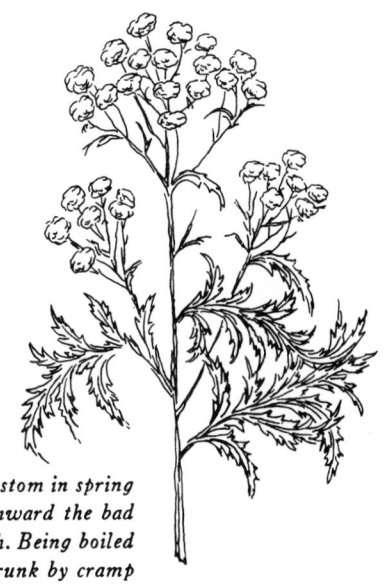

Tansy fried with eggs as is the custom in spring helpeth to digest and carry downward the bad humoure that trouble the stomach. Being boiled in oil it is good for the sinews shrunk by cramp or pained by cold.

CULPEPPER

At Easter a favorite dish was young leaves of tansy mixed with eggs. Here is a recipe dated 1420. "Take faire Tansy and grinde it in a mortar. Take eyern yolkes and whites and draw them through a streynour and straw al o the juice of the Tansy; and meddle the eggs and the juice togedre." This was fried in cakes and the herb was believed to be of value in purifying the body after a long winter diet of salt fish. Omelettes with the juice were called "tansy." In 1666 Samuel Pepys says he "spent an hour or two with her and ate a tansy." Tansy tea from the leaves, fresh or dried, was given for cramps, colic, gout, and even the plague. Here is a nice superstition from Sussex, England: the peasant will put tansy leaves in his shoe for the cure of ague. The herb is strongly scented with a bitter smell and taste and the flavor is not very pleasing to modern palates. However, in the Colonies, practically every farmyard had a clump of this aromatic medicinal herb. It was widely naturalized in New England by 1785 and is still fairly common along roadsides. Colonists picked the leaves before the plant blossomed to dye their wools a clear yellow.

Tarragon

Artemisia dracunculus
var. sativa
perennial to 2 feet

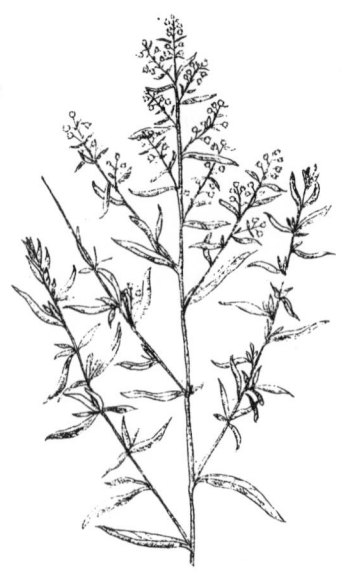

Tarragon is altogether used among other cold herbs, to temper their coldness, and they to temper its heat, so to give the better relish unto the sallet.

JOHN PARKINSON

Tarragon reached Europe from Asia in the Middle Ages. Charlemagne grew it under the name *draganeta*. Its name comes from the French word *esdragon*, meaning a little dragon. Some say it is named for the dragon-tail, serpentine coil of the roots and there is a legend that it sprang up along the serpent's track in the Garden of Eden. Since its origin the roots have been divided and shared because, unlike the wild tarragon, the garden variety does not set seeds.

An Arabian physician, Avicenna, 980–1037 A.D., used it as a medicine, and Elyot, an English doctor, wrote in 1538, "Tragonia has a taste like gungyr." Another writer of the sixteenth century says, "Tarragon is good in sallads with lettuce." Sir John Evelyn in 1693 says, "Tarragon is one of the perfumery or spicy furniture of our sallets." Culpepper adds that the leaves which are heating and drying are good for those that have the flux.

Thyme

Thymus vulgaris
perennial to 8 inches

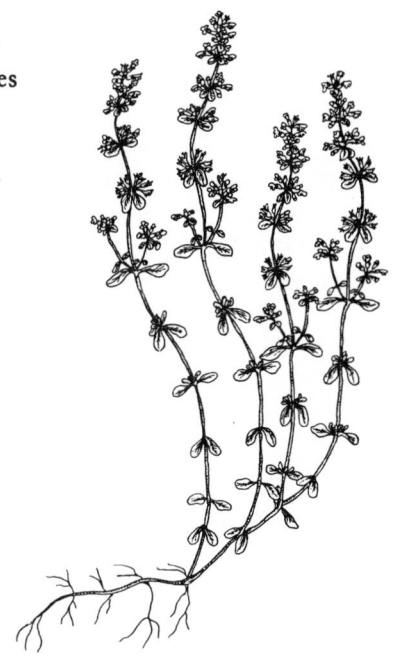

The thyme was on Sweet Mary's Bed
To bring her courage rare,
While Shepherds lifted up their hearts
In silent joyful prayer.

AUTHOR UNKNOWN

Theocritus in his *Idyls* speaks of "Thick growing thyme and roses wet with dew," and Virgil bespeaks its praises as does Horace. Sheep were taken to graze on fields of thyme to give their mutton a delightful flavor. Likewise, honey from thyme blossoms was especially prized.

Thyme is not mentioned in the north until about 1000 A.D. but was soon an established potherb in England. It was used widely in soups, sauces, and salads. Izaak Walton wanted it for his fish sauces and stuffings. In addition to its culinary uses, thyme was a valuable, fragrant, strewing herb. Later came its medicinal uses. Its oils had been extracted by 1725 in Germany and became an ingredient in many medicines. John Hill said in 1756, "Thyme is a better medicine for nervous cases than most that are used. The nightmare is a very troublesome disease and often puzzles the physician but it may be profitably cured by tea used from this plant." Earlier Culpepper had said, "Thyme is excellent good for those that are troubled with the gout. It easith pain in the loines and hips." It was considered good for the palsy, epilepsy, old coughs, and spitting of blood. It helped earache and toothache. It is still used in cough drops and to treat hookworms. "An infusion of thyme leaves removed the head ache occasioned by the debauch of the previous evening," wrote William Withering in the eighteenth century. This basic herb which filled so many needs was a "must" in Colonial gardens and was noted in New England by John Josselyn in his travels. Perhaps he knew that it was a favorite of the fairies in his native England; in fact if you wipe your eyes with it you can see the fairies.

Tulip

Tulipa
bulb 6 to 30 inches

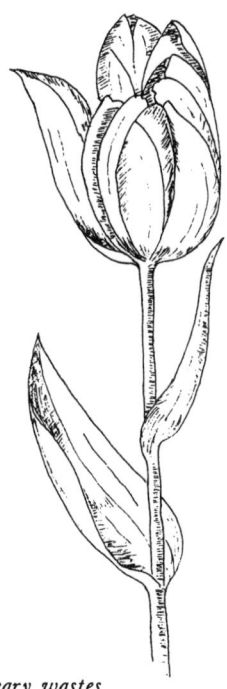

When o'er the cultur'd lawns and dreary wastes
Retiring Autumn flings her howling blasts . . .
Quick hears fair Tulipa the loud alarms
And folds her infant closer in her arms;
Soft plays affection round her bosom's throne,
And guards its life, forgetful of her own . . .

AUTHOR UNKNOWN

The name comes from a Persian word for turban referring to the shape of the inverted flower. Tulips were cultivated in Asia Minor for centuries before the colonial period in America. The Turks were the first to breed them in Europe. An Austrian ambassador to Constantinople took them to Vienna in 1554.

Later the Dutch became tulip specialists. "Tulipamania" swept Holland by 1638 when bulbs fetched fantastic prices before the market broke causing widespread bankruptcy. John Bartram in Philadelphia was sent "Tulip roots" by his friend Collinson from England in 1738. The Boston newspaper advertised fifty varieties for sale in 1760. The Colonial garden which could afford these treasures took particular pride and delight in their beauty. In reference to their value Stephen Blake's *Complete Gardners Practice,* 1664, tells how "To be revenged on a person who steals your tulips : sprinkle dry powdered Elecampane root on clove gilly flowers (dianthus) and give your flowers to the party that you desire to be revenged of, let it be a he or a she, they will delight in smelling to it, then they will draw this powder into their nostrels, which will make them fall a sneezing and a great trouble to the eyes, and by your leave will make the tears run down to their thighs." Here we find an early tear gas!

> *The tulip is the peacock among flowers; the one has no scent, the other no song; the one glories in its gown the other in its train.*
>
> FROM AN OLD FRENCH
> GARDENING BOOK

Violet

Viola odorata
perennial to 6 inches

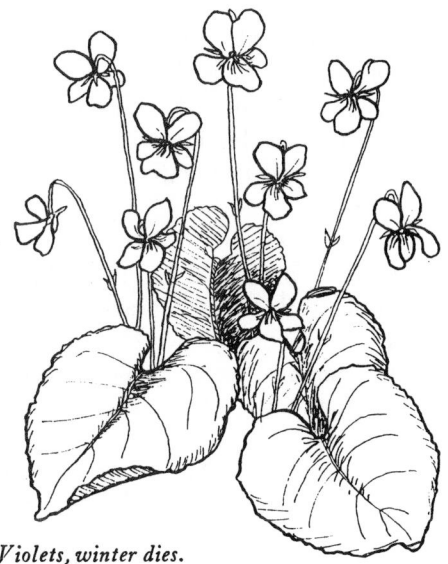

When wake the Violets, winter dies.
God does not send us strange flowers every year.
When the spring winds blow o'er the pleasant places,
The same dear things, lift up the same fair faces.
The violet is here.

Author Unknown

Violets were a great comfort to pioneer ladies. The
perennial violet, one of the many species of the viola
family, was at home in moist meadows, woodlands,
and gardens from Canada to the Carolinas. The name
is said to come from the Greek maiden, Ion or Io, for
whom violets were created when Zeus changed her into
a heifer to hide her from his jealous wife. Homer
and Virgil mentioned them often. They were used by
Athenians "to moderate anger, to procure sleep and to
comfort and strengthen the head." Pliny prescribes a
liniment of violet root and vinegar for gout and disorders of the spleen. He states that a garland of violets worn about the head will dispel the fumes of
wine and prevent headache and dizziness. In the Middle

Ages violets were considered powerful against "wicked spirytis." The violet in medieval flower symbolism signifies the humility of Our Lord. It was a culinary herb for salads and omelettes. Its medical uses were described in Bankes' *Herball* of 1525 in this way: "Heat oil of violet meddled with powder of poppy seed and anoint the small of the back therewith. . . . Also for him that may not sleep for sickness, seeth this herb well in water and at even let him soak well his feet in the water . . . and when he goeth to bed, bind this herb well to his temples."

It is surprising to us today that violets were both a culinary and a medicinal herb. We think of violets for their fragrance. In 1597 Gerard wrote, "The gallant grace of violets bring to a liberal and gentlemanly mind, the remembrance of honestie, comeliness and all kinds of virtues."

> *The excellence of the extract of violets above all other extracts is as the excellence of me above all the rest of creation.*
>
> *Attributed to* MOHAMMED

Winter Savory

Satureia montana
perennial to 15 inches

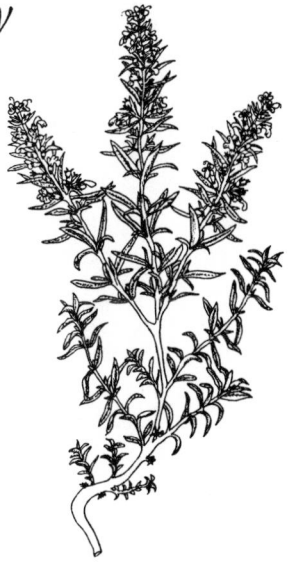

*Round their (the farmer's) houses let the
Cassis blossom grow, and the wild thyme with
its far flung sweetness, and a wealth of heavy
scented savory.*

VIRGIL, *Fourth Georgic*

Winter savory blooms from August to frost and is
much loved by bees. It flourished on Mount Atlas and
was called isope by the Greeks. The plant was taken
to Britain by the Romans and appears in many Saxon
recipes. It was used in the French *bouquet garni*, tied
into a cheesecloth bag with other herbs, and simmered
in soup and stewpots. It added flavor to meat dishes
and to trout. Drunk in wine Bankes' *Herball* says it
would "make thee a good meek stomach." It was one
of the herbs noted in New England by John Josselyn in
the eighteenth century so we know that our colonists
brought this old-time favorite from their homeland to
enjoy the flavor of its leaves and the beauty of its
flowers.

*Better is a dinner of herbs where love is than
a stalled ox and hatred therewith.*

Proverbs 15:17

67

Wormwood

Artemisia absinthium
subshrub to 4 feet

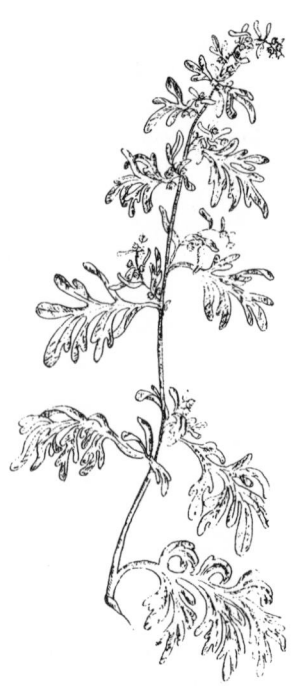

While wormwood hath seed get a handful of twaine
To save against March to make flea to refrain
When chamber is swept and wormwood is strown
No flea for his life dare abide to be known.

> TUSSER, *Five Points of*
> *Good Husbandry*

Wormwood is dedicated to Diana and is the symbol of bitterness. Legend has it that it sprang up in the track of the serpent when driven out of the Garden of Eden. It has been well known since 1500 B.C. Dioscorides' *Greek Herbal* in the first century declares it a remedy against intoxication. In Egypt it was used for headaches and to eliminate pinworms from the alimentary canal. It is still so used. In France in the Middle Ages midwives rubbed babies with the juice so they would never be cold or hot as long as they lived.

The colonists used wormwood to keep moths from clothing. Outward application relieved sprains and bruises. A conserve made from it relieved seasickness according to John Josselyn. The seeds kept fleas away and were powdered and sprinkled on books to prevent book lice. It was good to comfort the heart and to cleanse the stomach. If this herb were pounded and mixed with the gall of a bull and afterwards put into a man's eye, it took away all manner of impediments of sight.

Linnaeus (1707–78) said it was taken for liver complaint, scurvy, and gout. Brewers added the fruit of wormwood to their hops to make beer healthful. It is the base of absinth. It acts powerfully on the nerve centers, causing hallucinations, delirium, and sometimes insanity.

Yarrow

Achillea millefolium
perennial to 2 feet

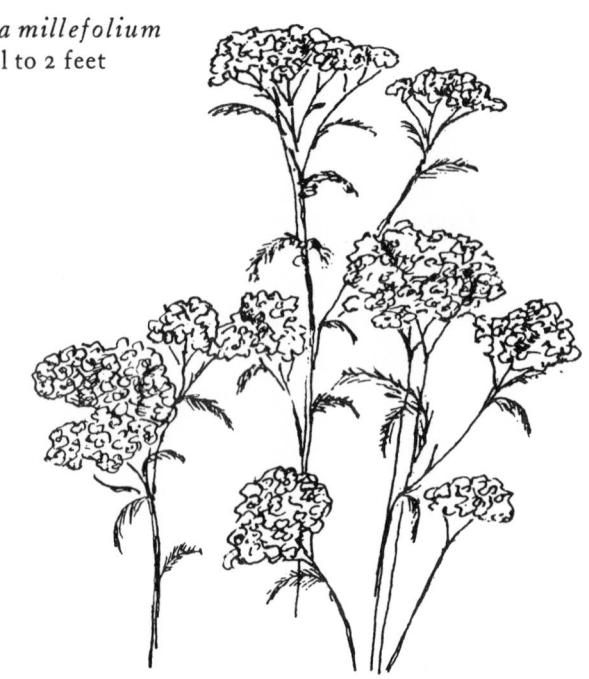

The Lord created medicines out of the earth
And a prudent man will have no disgust of them.

Ecclesiasticus

The white-flowering yarrow is a weed but its pink and red variety, roseum, is grown in gardens for its attractive flower clusters which bloom in May and June. The white, however, belongs in an herb garden and has been used since 1000 B.C. for agglutinating blood. Pliny says the name comes from Achilles who used it on his battlefields to stop the flow of blood in the arrow wounds of his men. The name yarrow comes from the Saxon *gearuwe*. It is also called nulfoil, starnch weed, noseblod, and sneezewort. It is native in Europe and Asia and was naturalized here at an early date. William Wood, who traveled in New England in 1629–66, spoke of "perennial yarrow" in gardens. Peter Kalm noted it in Philadelphia and Canada. For our pioneers it was a valuable medicine to stop bleeding in case of accidents. Housewives kept it on hand.

We leave the colonists with yarrow in their cupboards together with oils carefully distilled to ward off disease. Savory herbs are cooking in their soup pots. Dried herbs hang in their sheds. Fragrant ones put freshness in their homes. The dye pot hangs aside ready for the next length of woven cloth. How fortunate it was that the garden which provided so many necessities could furnish also solace for the soul.

> *Beds of all various herbs, for ever green,*
> *In beauteous order terminate the scene.*
>
> HOMER, quoted by
> HORACE WALPOLE in his
> *Essay on Modern Gardening*

Early Herbals Used for Drawings and Quotations

Bankes, Rycharde, *Herball,* 1525

Blackwell, Elizabeth, *A Curious Herbal* (2 vols.), 1739

Culpepper, Nicholas, *Complete Herbal,* 1649

Dioscorides, Pedanius, *The Greek Herbal,* first century A.D.

Fuchs, Leonhard, *Icones Plantarum,* 1545

Gerard, John, *The Herbal* or *General History of Plants*

Grieve, *A Modern Herbal*

Hill, John, *The British Herbal,* 1756

Matthiolus, Petorus Andreas, *Commentarii,* 1565

Parkinson, John, *Paradisi in Sole Paradisus Terrestris,* 1629

Tusser, Thomas, *Five Hundred Points of Good Husbandry,* 1597

Van de Passe, Crispian, *Hortus Floridus,* 1614

Index